Introduction

W ell, hello there, dear reader. You've just found your way into the world of chair yoga, which, I assure you, is heaps more exciting than it sounds. You're probably wondering why chair yoga exists, aren't you? Well, it's not because we wanted to give chairs something to do. It's not because we ran out of yoga mats. And it's not because we simply adore the sound of creaking furniture. No, chair yoga exists because it's the perfect bridge between the desire to maintain flexibility, strength, and balance, and the harsh reality of gravity pulling us down onto a soft, inviting chair.

Now, let's toss some laughter into the mix. Imagine combining that ha-ha-hilarious joke your friend told you last week with a chair pose. You know, the one that made you laugh so hard you nearly gave yourself a hernia? That's right, laughter and yoga are a match made in heaven, like peanut butter and jelly, like Netflix and weekends. It's about making your yoga practice not just a chore but a joy, a great time, a downright party.

And let's be real. There's a lot of hoopla out there about yoga being the golden ticket to weight loss. But as a nurse of 14 years and a yoga practitioner for 18 years, I can tell you this: Yoga isn't a magic pill. It won't magically melt away pounds while you sleep (though wouldn't that be fantastic?). It's a tool, a very powerful one, that when combined with a balanced diet and regular practice can help you lose weight, feel more energetic, and move better.

I am a strong advocate that yoga can be practiced by everyone! It does not require a certain body type, weight, size, or flexibility. I have worked with many private clients who have medical conditions and physical limitations. I have been able to create personalized yoga routines for them based on their unique needs. My goal is to show you how adaptive yoga can be. You don't have to let that bad knee or shoulder injury stop you from experiencing the benefits of a yoga practice.

So, what do you say? Are you ready to embark on this chair yoga adventure? It's going to be a wild ride, full of chair poses, belly laughs, and maybe a few chair creaks. But don't

THE JOY OF CHAIR YOGA FOR BEGINNERS AND SENIORS

LOSE WEIGHT, MOVE FREELY, FEEL MORE ENERGETIC, AND HAVE SOME LAUGHS!

HEATHER DOLSON, R.N., BScN

HEATHER ON HEALTH

CONTENTS

worry, I've got your back... and your knees... and your hips. Now, let's get started, shall we?

CHAPTER ONE

CHAIR YOGA: WHAT'S THE BIG IDEA?

D id you know that your trusty armchair could double as your new fitness partner? Yes, you heard it right! That comfy recliner, the silent observer of your TV binges, and the ultimate refuge after a long day, has a secret superhero identity. It's a yoga mat, a personal trainer, and a wellness coach, all rolled into one! Welcome, my friend, to the surprisingly sprightly world of chair yoga.

The ABCs of Chair Yoga

Before we start twisting and stretching, let's establish some ground rules. No, I'm not about to tell you to stop eating cookies and chips, although you might want to put that cookie down for a moment. Also, a treat is nice every once in a while. When it comes to nutrition, I am a strong advocate for everything in moderation. If you're going to indulge in the donut or chocolate cupcake, do so fully and enjoy it! Let's get acquainted with the basic principles and poses of chair yoga. We will dive deeper into these poses later on.

Armchair Warrior Pose:

The Warrior Pose in traditional yoga is all about strength and endurance. But here, you won't be standing on one leg or engaging in a battle with gravity. Instead, you'll be sitting tall in your chair, feet firmly planted on the ground, and engaging your core muscles as you stretch your arms out. Think of it as your 'I've got this' pose, preparing you for the challenges ahead, be it a yoga session or handling stress in life.

Seated Mountain Pose:

Mountain Pose is about grounding and stability in traditional yoga. In its chair version, you sit upright, feet flat on the ground, hands resting on your thighs. It's like being a mountain, steady and unshakeable. Only instead of braving winds and storms, you're facing the perils of this adventure we call life!

Chair Pigeon Pose:

The Pigeon Pose is a hip opener in traditional yoga, and in the chair version, it's less about cooing like a pigeon and more about stretching those hip muscles. But feel free to coo! You'll be sitting upright, one foot on the floor, and the other ankle resting on the opposite knee. It's like crossing your legs, only with a bit more oomph.

Revolved Chair Pose:

The Revolved Chair Pose is a seated twist where you rotate your upper body to one side while keeping your lower body stable. Think of it as a gentle wringing out of your spine, like you would wring out a wet towel, only much gentler.

Chair Savasana:

Savasana or Corpse Pose is usually the final pose in a yoga session, meant for relaxation and integration. In the chair version, you'll sit comfortably, close your eyes, and let your body relax fully into the chair. It's like taking a power nap, just without the snoring.

Now that we've met our main players, let's talk a bit more about chair yoga as a practice.

Chair Yoga: The Inclusive Fitness Revolution

Chair yoga is a modified version of traditional yoga that brings the benefits of this ancient practice to those who may have mobility limitations, are recovering from injuries, or just happen to love their chairs a little too much. It's yoga that adapts to you, not the other way around.

The need for chair yoga stems from a very simple realization: Yoga, with its promise of holistic wellness, should be accessible to everyone. And when I say everyone, I mean everyone - from the sprightly 25-year-old who can touch their toes without breaking a sweat, to the wise 85-year-old who considers it a victory to put on their socks in the morning.

So, whether you're a senior citizen seeking to add a little flexibility to your golden years, a busy professional looking for stress relief between Zoom meetings, or a complete beginner who thinks 'Downward Dog' is a sequel to 'Reservoir Dogs', chair yoga has something for you.

In the next chapters, we'll delve deeper into the world of chair yoga, debunking myths, addressing concerns, and shedding light on its potential for weight loss. But for now, let's revel in the fact that your chair isn't just for sitting anymore. It's your stepping stone to better health, improved flexibility, and a whole lot of fun. So, are you ready to give your chair the upgrade it deserves? Let's get started on this chair yoga adventure!

Why Chair Yoga is a Game Changer

"No pain, no gain" - you've likely heard this age-old adage before, especially in the context of fitness and exercise. But what if I told you that you could make significant gains without the associated pain? That's where chair yoga steals the spotlight.

Gentle on Joints

With each passing year, our bodies naturally undergo changes. Some of these changes are more visible, like the appearance of grey hairs or wrinkles, while others are less noticeable but equally impactful. One such change is the gradual wear and tear of our joints.

Now, imagine a workout routine that not only respects this inevitable decline in joint health but also helps to alleviate the associated discomfort. Chair yoga, with its gentle and low-impact movements, is kind to your joints. It is gentler and allows you to find your own body language with a soothing, joint-friendly exercise alternative.

Improves Balance

It's not just about being able to walk a tightrope or perform a flawless pirouette. Balance plays a critical role in our daily activities, from walking up a flight of stairs to reaching for that top shelf in the kitchen. As we age, maintaining balance can become a bit more challenging, increasing the risk of falls.

Enter chair yoga. With poses that emphasize stability and core strength, chair yoga is like a personal balance trainer. This practice can become an invisible safety net, providing you with the confidence to navigate your daily activities with less fear of falling.

Boosts Flexibility

If you've ever experienced the frustration of not being able to tie your shoelaces or pick up a dropped item because of stiffness, you'll appreciate the value of flexibility. Chair yoga, with its array of stretches and poses, helps to increase your range of motion. It's as if you're gently coaxing your muscles and joints out of their comfort zones, encouraging them to become more flexible and accommodating.

Enhances Strength

In chair yoga, your own body weight serves as the perfect resistance tool, helping to build strength without the need for dumbbells or resistance bands. Each pose is like a mini power-lifting session for your muscles, helping to enhance strength and endurance.

Promotes Relaxation and Mindfulness

In the hustle and bustle of modern life, moments of relaxation can be hard to come by. Chair yoga, with its emphasis on mindful breathing and conscious movement, offers an oasis of calm. Allow your chair yoga practice to be a bubble of tranquility, away from the noise and chaos of the outside world, if only for a few moments.

Maintain Muscle Tone

Just as an unused engine can rust over time, unused muscles can lose their tone and definition. Chair yoga helps to keep your muscles active and engaged, preserving their tone and function. Think of it as a tune-up for your muscles, helping to keep them running smoothly.

Reduces Stress and Improves Mood

Life can throw curveballs that leave us feeling stressed and overwhelmed. Chair yoga serves as a defense mechanism against these stressors, helping to lower stress levels and improve mood.

Improves Sleep Quality and Enhances Overall Quality of Life

Tossing and turning at night can leave you feeling drained and lethargic during the day. Chair yoga, with its relaxing and stress-busting properties, can help improve sleep quality. We will cover mindful breathing techniques that you can implement the next time you're lying there at 3 a.m. looping around worrisome thoughts.

Moreover, regular practice of chair yoga can have a ripple effect on your overall quality of life. From boosting your energy levels to enhancing your physical function, chair yoga touches every aspect of well-being. When you can make this a part of your daily routine, you will be amazed at how the simplicity of it will add a spark of vitality and joy.

So, there you have it. Chair yoga isn't just about doing yoga on a chair. It's a fitness revolution that caters to you, regardless of your age or fitness level. It respects your individuality and is designed to your unique needs, making it a truly inclusive form of exercise. Now, aren't you excited to see what wonders chair yoga has in store for you? Let's continue this exciting exploration in the next chapter!

Your Chair is Your New Best Friend

Let's face it; your chair is already an integral part of your daily routine. It's there when you enjoy your morning coffee, engrossed in a thrilling novel, or when you're simply unwinding after a long day. But who knew this humble piece of furniture could also play a significant role in your fitness journey?

No Fancy Equipment Needed

When starting a new fitness routine, one of the biggest deterrents can be the long list of equipment you're told you need - dumbbells, resistance bands, yoga mats, stability balls, the list can be endless. And let's not even start on the cost and the space they occupy in your home. But what if your fitness routine required nothing more than an everyday object you already own?

That's right! With chair yoga, all you need is a sturdy chair, and you're good to go. No more tripping over dumbbells or struggling to store bulky exercise equipment. This simplicity not only makes chair yoga wallet-friendly but also eliminates any stress related to setting up for your workout. It's time to look at your favorite chair with newfound respect!

Exercise Anywhere, Anytime

The beauty of chair yoga lies in its versatility. Whether you're in the comfort of your living room, at your office desk, or even waiting for a flight at the airport, your chair-based fitness routine can accompany you. No more scheduling woes or skipped workouts because you can't make it to the gym.

Remember those endless TV commercial breaks that used to annoy you? Now, they can become your mini-chair yoga sessions. Or how about that hour-long conference call? Just turn off your camera, and you have a stealthy chair yoga workout right there. With chair yoga, you have the flexibility to weave in a fitness routine into your day, no matter how packed it might be.

Comfort and Stability

Let's be honest; traditional yoga poses can sometimes feel like you're trying to twist your body into a pretzel. It can be daunting, especially for beginners and seniors who might not have the flexibility or balance they once did. That's where chair yoga shines.

Your chair serves as a supportive prop, providing the stability you need to perform a variety of yoga poses with confidence and ease. Plus, there's the added advantage of being able to sit down whenever you need a break. Trust me, your back and knees will thank you!

Chair yoga is about making fitness accessible, uncomplicated, and enjoyable. It's about breaking down the barriers that often discourage us from adopting a healthy lifestyle. So, the next time you cozy up in your favorite chair, remember, it's not just a chair. It's your new best friend on your wellness journey, always ready to support you, one yoga pose at a time.

As you continue reading, you'll discover more about the versatility and adaptability of chair yoga, and how it can be customized to suit your needs, preferences, and fitness goals. From debunking common misconceptions to exploring the potential for weight loss, you're about to see your humble chair in a whole new light. But for now, give your chair a pat, and let's get ready to dive deeper into the world of chair yoga. Your adventure is just beginning!

Addressing Misconceptions: Chair Yoga is Not Boring

Now, let's address the elephant in the room. Some folks believe that chair yoga is just a tad too easy or, dare we say, dull. If you're one of those who think that chair yoga is a snooze-fest, prepare to have your mind blown.

First off, chair yoga is not a walk in the park (unless, of course, you're doing it at the park!). It can be as gentle or as sweat-inducing as you make it. The secret lies in tuning into your body's messages and adjusting the poses to match your comfort and ability. Remember, your body is the boss here, and it calls the shots.

The beauty of chair yoga lies in its variety each serving up its unique flavor of benefits. And before you ask, no, you won't be stuck doing the same three poses over and over. Chair yoga offers an extensive menu of poses and sequences that will keep your practice fresh and exciting.

Take the Sun Salutation sequence, for example. This sequence is the bread and butter of many traditional yoga practices, and guess what? It can be adapted for the chair. That's right! You can get a full-body workout, improving your strength, flexibility, and balance, all from the comfort of your chair.

But wait, there's more! Chair yoga is not just about the physical poses. It's about the experience, the connection you forge with your body and mind. It's about cultivating mindfulness, staying present, and being engaged in every pose. It's like having a heart-to-heart conversation with your body, understanding its needs, its limitations, and its potential.

This focus on mindfulness makes each chair yoga session a unique experience. You know when you really enjoy something and you get so completely engrossed in the activity that you lose track of time? And just like that, boredom gets booted out of the window.

Moreover, the beauty of chair yoga lies in its adaptability. Each pose can be modified to suit your comfort level, keeping the practice challenging yet enjoyable. You can progress at your own pace, gradually increasing the intensity of the poses as your strength and flexibility improve.

Chair yoga is anything but boring. It's a dynamic, adaptable, and engaging practice that respects your individuality and caters to your unique needs. It's a practice that challenges you, supports you, and most importantly, grows with you. And who knows? You might just find yourself looking forward to your chair yoga sessions more than your favorite TV show. Now, wouldn't that be something?

Now, let's talk about something that's on everyone's mind - weight loss. Can chair yoga help you shed those stubborn pounds? Is it possible to get a good workout while sitting down? Can you really get fit with chair yoga? Stick around, because we're about to dive into the weight loss potential of chair yoga. Spoiler alert: You're in for a pleasant surprise!

The Weight Loss Potential of Chair Yoga

So, you're probably thinking: "Can I really lose weight while sitting?" It sounds too good to be true, right? But let's unravel this mystery. Chair yoga, in all its seated glory, holds a promising potential for weight loss. And let me assure you; it's not about sweating buckets or starving yourself. It's a more holistic and sustainable approach to weight loss.

The Calorie-Burning Chair

Now, before you roll your eyes, let me clarify. Chair yoga isn't going to burn calories like a high-intensity spinning class or a grueling boot camp session. But that's not the point. Chair yoga aims to provide a gentle, low-impact exercise option that can contribute to your overall calorie-burning endeavors.

In each chair yoga session, you're moving and stretching your body, using your muscles, and increasing your heart rate. All of these activities require energy, which means you're burning calories. Your body is a calorie-burning machine, only at a slower and more sustainable pace.

The Mind-Body Connection

But chair yoga's potential for weight loss isn't just about the physical aspects. It's also about the connection between your mind and body. When you practice chair yoga, you're not just moving your body; you're also bringing your attention to your breath, your movements, and your body's responses.

This increased mindfulness can have a profound impact on your relationship with food. You become more aware of your hunger and fullness cues, helping you to eat more intuitively. You start to notice how certain foods make you feel, allowing you to make healthier choices.

In other words, chair yoga can help you swap mindless munching for mindful eating.

Stress Less, Weigh Less

Let's not forget the stress-busting benefits of chair yoga. Stress is often a significant contributor to weight gain. When we're stressed, we're more likely to reach for comfort foods, skip our workouts, and have trouble sleeping.

Chair yoga, with its relaxing poses and deep breathing exercises, serves as a natural stress reliever helping you unwind and de-stress. And when you're less stressed, you're more likely to make healthier choices, sleep better, and maintain a balanced weight.

In a nutshell, chair yoga supports weight loss by providing a gentle, calorie-burning workout, promoting mindful eating, and reducing stress. It's not a quick fix or a magic solution, but a sustainable and holistic approach to weight loss.

So, the next time you take a seat, remember that you're not just resting. You're stepping into a world of possibilities, where weight loss doesn't require punishing workouts or restrictive diets. You're embracing a kinder, gentler approach to weight loss, one chair pose at a time.

Ready to explore more about chair yoga? Hold tight to your chair handles, because we're just getting started! In the upcoming chapters, we'll dive deeper into the world of chair yoga, exploring its various poses, how to adapt them to your needs, and how to incorporate them into your daily routine. So, stay seated, because the best is yet to come!

No Pain, All Gain: The Gentle Power of Chair Yoga

You've probably heard the saying, "No pain, no gain." It's a common mantra in the fitness world, suggesting that you have to endure discomfort or even pain to see results. But what if you could gain without the pain? What if you could get fit, flexible, and strong without wincing, grunting, or gasping for breath? That's where chair yoga steps in, promising gains without the pain. Let's take a closer look at how chair yoga makes this possible.

Low Impact, High Results

Traditional workouts often involve a lot of jumping, lunging, and lifting, which can be hard on your joints. Chair yoga, on the other hand, is a low-impact exercise that's gentle on your joints, but still offers impressive results.

Think of it this way: chair yoga is more subtle like a gentle breeze that cools you down on a hot day, but the relief it brings is undeniable. Similarly, chair yoga might not have you panting or sweating like a high-intensity workout, but it still works your muscles, enhances your flexibility, and improves your balance.

Safe for All Fitness Levels

One of the significant advantages of chair yoga is its accessibility. Whether you're an exercise newbie or a seasoned fitness enthusiast, chair yoga is safe for all fitness levels.

I want you to enjoy the dance of life. There is no one else you have to keep up with. You get to dance your own dance at your own pace and to your own beat. That's what chair yoga is like. It's like your own dance that you can do, regardless of age, mobility, or fitness level.

Customizable to Individual Needs

Perhaps the most beautiful thing about chair yoga is its adaptability. You can modify the poses to suit your comfort level, making the practice uniquely yours.

You can pick and choose the poses that work best for you, making your practice as satisfying and fulfilling to your unique needs.

Chair yoga is a fitness approach that cares about your comfort and respects your limitations. It doesn't ask you to be anything other than what you are. It's a nod to the fact that fitness isn't a one-size-fits-all concept, but a personal journey that should be tailored to your unique needs and abilities.

So, the next time you sit down in your favorite chair, remember, that it's not just a resting spot. It's a gateway to better fitness, improved health, and a happier you. So, recline, relax, and get ready to redefine what it means to sit!

Remember, the key to unlocking the full potential of chair yoga lies in understanding its principles, embracing its versatility, and appreciating its simplicity. Every pose, every breath, every moment you spend in your chair can contribute to your wellness journey. So, why wait? Your chair is ready, and so are you. Let's turn the ordinary into the extraordinary.

Chapter Two

How to Speak Yoga

Let's face it, stepping into a yoga class for the first time can feel a bit like landing on an alien planet. There's the strange language, the unusual movements, and people twisting their bodies in ways you've only seen in pretzels. But don't worry dear reader, you've got a trusty guide by your side. In this chapter, we'll decode the mysterious language of yoga, one funny-sounding word at a time.

You see, yoga isn't just about bending and stretching. It's also about connecting with a centuries-old tradition that comes with its own unique vocabulary. Learning this lingo is like learning a secret handshake. It's your ticket to feel more at home in the world of yoga, and more importantly, in your own body. So, let's roll out our imaginary yoga mats and dive into the ABCs of yoga language.

Deciphering Yoga Lingo

Let's start with four fundamental terms in the yoga world: Asana, Pranayama, Namaste, and Sat Nam. These terms are the bread and butter of any yoga practice, and understanding them will give you a solid foundation to build upon.

Asana: The Fancy Word for Pose

In yoga, every movement or position you make with your body is called an 'Asana.' It's a Sanskrit word that translates to 'pose' or 'posture.' You can think of Asanas as the different dance moves in the choreography of a yoga practice. Some are gentle and slow, like a waltz, while others are more dynamic and challenging, like a salsa.

Each Asana has its own name, often inspired by nature. For instance, *Tadasana* or Mountain Pose, where you stand tall and grounded, mimicking the stillness and strength of a mountain. Or *Vrikshasana* or Tree Pose, where you balance on one foot, with your other foot resting on the inner thigh of the standing leg, much like a tree stands rooted to the ground.

So the next time you're in a chair yoga session and you hear the instructor say, "Let's move into our next Asana," know that it's your cue to strike a pose!

Pranayama: The Art of Breathing

Pranayama may sound like a fancy tropical fruit, but it's actually all about the breath. The term '*Pranayama*' is derived from two Sanskrit words: 'Prana,' which means life force or breath, and 'Yama,' which means control. So, *Pranayama* is essentially the practice of controlling your breath.

Think of *Pranayama* as the music that accompanies your dance of Asanas. It sets the rhythm and pace of your movements, helping to create harmony between your body and mind. Different *Pranayama* techniques can either energize you, like a catchy pop song or calm you down, like a soothing lullaby.

For example, there's the '*Ujjayi*' or 'Victorious' breath, where you breathe in and out through your nose, creating a gentle sound, like the waves of the ocean. It's often used during yoga practice to help stay focused and grounded.

Remember, in chair yoga, your breath is your ally. It guides you, supports you, and most importantly, reminds you to keep going, one breath at a time.

Namaste: More Than Just a Greeting

You've probably heard this term before, perhaps as a greeting or a sign-off at the end of a yoga class. '*Namaste*' is a traditional Indian salutation that means 'I bow to you.' It's a way of acknowledging the divinity within all of us.

Saying '*Namaste*' is kind of like giving someone a warm hug without the physical contact. It's a way of expressing respect and connection, not just to the person you're greeting, but to the entire universe.

In chair yoga, saying '*Namaste'* is like adding a cherry on top of your practice. It's a moment of gratitude – for your body, for the chair supporting you, and for the opportunity to experience the benefits of yoga.

Sat Nam: A Mantra of Truth

Chanting or saying '*Sat Nam*' comes from Kundalini yoga. '*Sat*' rhymes with "but" and '*Nam*' rhymes with "calm." *Sat Nam* means "Truth is my Identity" or "I am Truth." We say it as a greeting or at the end of a class. It is used in many kriyas and meditations. *Kriya* is just another word for a specific sequence of exercises.

Congratulations! You're now well-versed in four fundamental terms of yoga lingo. You've learned that an '*Asana*' is not a type of pasta, '*Pranayama*' is not a tropical fruit, and '*Namaste*' and '*Sat Nam*' are more than just a fancy way of saying hello.

This is just the beginning of your yoga vocabulary journey. Up ahead, we have more funny yoga words to explore and some that even sound like desserts. So, keep your curiosity alight, and let's continue this linguistic adventure.

Funny Yoga Words You'll Love

We've covered the basics of yoga lingo, and now it's time to add a dash of humor to our linguistic lesson. Yes, yoga can be serious, profound, and philosophical, but it can also be downright funny. So, let's dive right in and explore some yoga terms that, despite their serious undertones, can't help but make us chuckle.

Savasana: The Nap Pose

First on our list is *Savasana*. Now, if you've ever secretly wished for a nap in the middle of an exercise routine, you're in for a treat. *Savasana*, also known as the Corpse Pose (I know, a bit morbid, but stay with me here), is essentially a well-deserved nap after your yoga practice.

You've just completed a series of chair yoga poses, your muscles are humming with newfound energy, and your mind is buzzing with a sense of achievement. What better way to wrap up your session than with a peaceful nap, right? That's precisely what *Savasana* offers.

In *Savasana*, you sit comfortably in your chair, close your eyes, and let your body relax. You're not just chilling out; you're also allowing your body to absorb the benefits of the poses you've just performed. So, the next time you're yearning for a quick snooze, remember, it's not laziness, it's *Savasana*.

Chaturanga: The Yoga Push-Up

Next on our laughter list is *Chaturanga*, a term that might remind you of a catchy Latin dance number. But in the yoga world, *Chaturanga* is often referred to as the yoga push-up. Yes, you heard that right. Yoga has its own version of the classic push-up.

Now, you might be wondering how on earth you're supposed to do a push-up while sitting in a chair. Well, that's where the magic of chair yoga comes in. In chair yoga, *Chaturanga* can be modified into a seated push-up. You'd place your hands on the armrests of the chair and engage your core as you lift your body off the seat, using your arms for support. It's like a push-up, only without the face-planting risk.

So, the next time you're doing a chair yoga session, and you hear the term *Chaturanga*, don't break into a dance. Instead, brace yourself for some arm-strengthening action.

Vinyasa: The Yoga Dance

Last, but not least, we have *Vinyasa*, a term that sounds like it could be the name of a trendy new smoothie. But in yoga lingo, *Vinyasa* is all about flow. It's a sequence of poses that are performed in sync with your breath, creating a dance-like rhythm.

Think of *Vinyasa* as a choreographed dance routine. You move from one pose to another, each movement flowing into the next, guided by the rhythm of your breath. It's like your body is swaying to its own inner music, creating a sense of harmony and fluidity.

In chair yoga, *Vinyasa* could involve a sequence of seated poses, like a seated sun salutation, where you move from a seated mountain pose to a seated forward bend, to a seated cobra pose, all in one smooth flow.

Yoga isn't just about striking poses and holding your breath. It's a living, breathing, and occasionally hilarious practice that can bring joy, health, and a whole lot of laughter into your life. Remember, it's not the perfection of the poses that matters, but the joy of the journey. So, keep practicing, keep laughing, and most importantly, keep enjoying this wonderful practice called chair yoga.

In the upcoming sections, we'll continue to explore the fun and fascinating world of yoga lingo. So, keep that curiosity brewing, because there's a lot more to discover. From yoga terms that sound like desserts to understanding the deeper meaning behind these terms, we've got a lot more ground to cover. So, sit tight, and let's continue this linguistic adventure.

Yoga Terms That Sound Like Desserts

Alright, it's time to serve up some yoga terms that sound like they belong on a dessert menu. If the thought of exercise makes you crave something sweet, then you're in for a real treat.

Bakasana: Crow Pose, Not a Bakery Item

First on our list is *Bakasana*, which sounds like it could be a flaky pastry fresh out of the oven. But before you reach for the oven mitts, let's set the record straight. *Bakasana*, in yoga lingo, is known as the Crow Pose.

This balancing posture requires strength, flexibility, and a dash of bravery, much like trying to bake a soufflé for the first time. In its full form, you balance on your hands with your knees tucked into your armpits, resembling a crow perched on a branch.

Now, if you're wondering how to do this while seated, don't fret! In chair yoga, you can mimic the Crow Pose by lifting one foot off the ground at a time, engaging your core, and finding your balance. You won't exactly resemble a crow, but you'll definitely give your muscles a scrumptious workout!

Tadasana: Mountain Pose, Not a Tapioca Pudding

Next up is *Tadasana,* a term that might remind you of a creamy tapioca pudding. But instead of indulging in a sweet treat, you'll be channeling the strength and stability of a mountain.

Indeed, *Tadasana*, or Mountain Pose, is all about grounding yourself and finding stillness, much like a mountain standing tall amidst the changing seasons. In chair yoga, you can practice *Tadasana* by sitting up straight, feet firmly on the ground, and hands resting on your thighs. It's a simple pose, yet it can make you feel grounded and centered, just like enjoying a comforting bowl of tapioca pudding!

Sukhasana: Easy Pose, Not a Sugar Rush

Last on our dessert menu is *Sukhasana*, which sounds like it could be a sweet burst of flavors in your mouth. However, in the world of yoga, *Sukhasana* refers to the Easy Pose, better known as a cross-legged posture when on the floor.

Don't let the name fool you, though. The Easy Pose isn't about taking it easy or slacking off. It's a sitting posture that encourages a straight spine, relaxed shoulders, and a quiet mind. It's the ideal pose for meditation or for those moments when you need a break from your day, much like savoring a piece of your favorite chocolate.

In chair yoga, you can achieve *Sukhasana* by sitting comfortably in your chair, feet flat on the floor, and hands resting on your thighs. It's a pose that invites calmness and relaxation, offering a sweet respite from the hustle and bustle of life.

You've just added three dessert-like yoga terms to your vocabulary. So, the next time you hear these words, remember, that they're not about satisfying your sweet tooth, but about enriching your chair yoga practice.

As we continue to explore the delightful world of chair yoga, remember to savor each pose, each breath, and each moment, much like you'd savor a delicious dessert. After all, chair yoga isn't just about getting fit and losing weight; it's about experiencing joy, laughter, and maybe even a little bit of sweetness along the way. So, let's keep this banquet of knowledge going because the best is yet to come!

Isn't it amazing how much fun we're having learning about chair yoga? We're not only getting healthier, but we're also expanding our vocabulary and having a few giggles along the way. So, let's keep this momentum going. Up next, we'll be diving into one of the most crucial aspects of chair yoga - breathing. So, take a deep breath, and let's continue this exciting adventure.

Chapter Three

Breathe In, Breathe Out

The Lifeline of Chair Yoga

It's a truth universally acknowledged that we humans can't live without air. But did you know there's a whole lot more to breathing than just keeping us alive? Let's pause for a moment and consider something we do around 20,000 times a day without even thinking about it – breathing. It's automatic, effortless, and yet, when harnessed correctly, can transform our chair yoga experience from good to absolutely fantastic!

If chair yoga were a symphony, your breath would be the conductor, guiding each pose, setting the rhythm, and bringing harmony to your practice. But how exactly does something as simple as inhaling and exhaling hold such profound power? Let's unravel this mystery, one breath at a time.

The Importance of Inhaling and Exhaling

Oxygenates the Body

The act of breathing in (inhaling) draws oxygen into your lungs, which is then transported by the bloodstream to every cell in your body. As you breathe out (exhale), your body gets rid of carbon dioxide, a waste gas that your body doesn't need. Think of it as your body's very own recycling program, continuously supplying fresh oxygen while disposing of unwanted waste.

As we practice chair yoga, this oxygen supply to the body becomes even more critical. The yoga poses and movements we perform require energy, and oxygen plays a crucial role in producing this energy. So, when we breathe deeply, we're essentially fueling our yoga practice, providing our muscles with the energy they need to stretch, strengthen, and balance.

Calms the Mind

You've probably noticed that when you're stressed or anxious, your breath becomes shallow and rapid. This type of breathing can trigger a 'fight or flight' response, making you feel more anxious. On the flip side, deep, slow breathing can help to calm your mind, triggering a relaxation response in your body.

Here's where chair yoga comes in. As we move through the yoga poses, we're encouraged to focus on our breath, to inhale deeply, and to exhale fully. This focus on deep, mindful breathing can have a calming effect on the mind, helping to reduce stress and promote a sense of peace and calm. It's like giving your mind a mini vacation, a temporary escape from the hustle and bustle of life.

Enhances Yoga Practice

Now, you might be thinking, "But I breathe all the time. How is breathing in chair yoga any different?" The difference lies in the conscious control of the breath. In our day-to-day life, we often take shallow breaths, barely using our lung capacity. In chair yoga, we learn to breathe deeply, filling our lungs with fresh air on each inhale and fully emptying them on each exhale.

This deep, conscious breathing can enhance our chair yoga practice in several ways. It helps us to move more mindfully, to hold the poses longer, and to stay focused during our practice. It's like having an inner guide, leading us through our practice one breath at a time.

So, the next time you're doing chair yoga, remember to breathe. Not just the automatic, barely-there kind of breathing, but deep, conscious, belly-filling breathing. Notice how it oxygenates your body, calms your mind, and enhances your practice. It's not just about filling your lungs with air; it's about filling your practice with life, one breath at a time.

As we continue our exploration of chair yoga, we'll learn more about the role of breath in our practice. We'll discover fun breathing exercises that don't involve balloons, and learn how to breathe like a baby again. So, stay tuned, keep breathing, and let's continue this exciting journey into the world of chair yoga.

Fun Breathing Exercises That Don't Involve Balloons

Belly Breathing

Say hello to belly breathing, the superstar of the breathing world. No, it's not about making your belly look like a balloon (although it does involve a bit of inflation and deflation). It's about learning to breathe deeply into your belly, using your diaphragm to its full potential.

To give this a whirl, find a comfy spot on your chair. Make sure your feet are flat on the ground. Sit up as straight as possible. Rest your hands on your belly, as though it's a precious crystal ball. Now, as you breathe in, imagine filling this ball with fresh, cleansing air. Feel your belly rise under your hands as the crystal ball inside expands. As you breathe out, let your belly gently fall, releasing the air from your imaginary crystal ball.

This simple act of belly breathing can work wonders on your chair yoga practice. It helps you to stay focused, moves your breath deeper into your body, and even gives your abdominal muscles a mini workout.

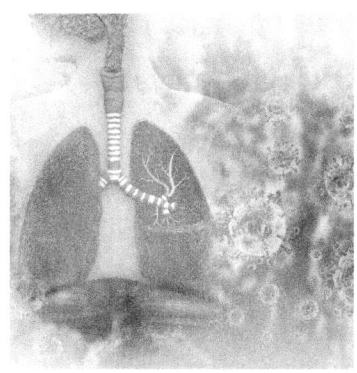

Box Breathing

Next up, we have box breathing, also known as square breathing. No, it's not about turning your breath into a box. It's about creating a rhythmic pattern with your breath, just like the four equal sides of a box.

To practice box breathing, picture a box in your mind. Now, each side of the box will represent a count of four. As you breathe in, count to four (that's the first side of the box). Hold your breath for a count of four (that's the second side). Then, breathe out for a count of four (there goes the third side), and finally, hold your breath again for a count of four (and that's the last side of the box).

Box breathing is like giving your breath a steady rhythm to dance to. It can help to calm your mind, slow your heart rate, and even improve your mood. So, the next time you're feeling frazzled, just remember your box. It's a simple yet effective way to add a little tranquility to your day.

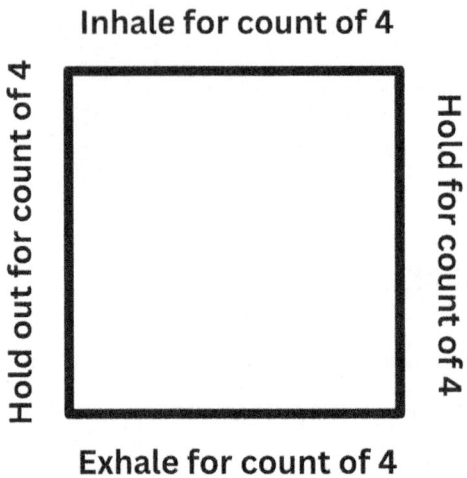

Lion's Breath

Last but not least, let's get a little wild with Lion's Breath. Don't worry, it's not about roaring like a lion (although there is a bit of roaring involved). It's about releasing tension, letting go of stress, and, most importantly, having a bit of fun!

To try Lion's Breath, sit tall in your chair, take a deep breath in, and as you breathe out, open your mouth wide, stick out your tongue, and let out a roaring sigh. Don't be shy; let your inner lion roar!

Lion's Breath is a fantastic way to release stress, stretch your facial muscles, and bring a little lightheartedness to your chair yoga practice. Plus, it's a great excuse to make faces and let loose. So, go ahead, channel your inner lion, and let the world hear you roar!

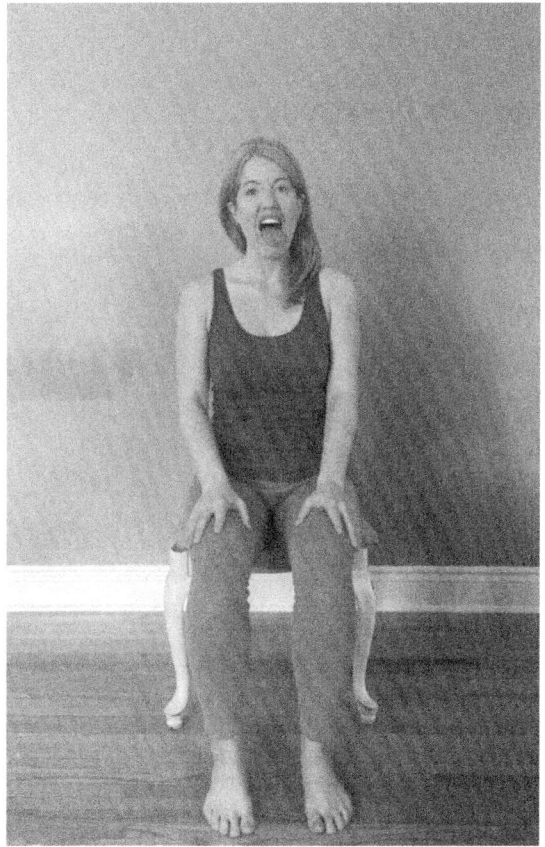

Lion's Breath

So now you are equipped with three fun and effective breathing exercises to jazz up your chair yoga practice. Whether you're connecting with your core with belly breathing, finding tranquility with box breathing, or unleashing your inner lion, remember, it's all about the breath. So, breathe deep, breathe with intention, and most importantly, have fun with your breath!

How to Breathe Like a Baby Again

Diaphragmatic Breathing

Ever watched a baby while they're peacefully snoozing? You'll notice their little tummy rising and falling with each breath. That's diaphragmatic breathing, a natural and highly efficient way of breathing that we're all born with. But as we grow older, stress, poor posture, and a hurried lifestyle often lead us away from this natural rhythm, towards shallow, chest-based breathing.

To reclaim this baby-like breathing pattern, let's try some diaphragmatic breathing. Sit comfortably in your chair, place one hand on your chest and the other on your belly. Now, take a slow, deep breath, pulling the air right down into your belly. You should feel the hand on your belly rise, while the hand on your chest remains still. Exhale gently, feeling your belly fall. It's like pumping air into a balloon and then letting it out slowly.

Practicing diaphragmatic breathing during your chair yoga sessions can help reduce stress, improve oxygenation, and enhance your overall practice. It's like returning to your roots, breathing like a baby, carefree and natural.

Humming Bee Breath

From babies, let's move on to bees. We're talking about a fun and soothing breathing technique called the Humming Bee Breath or 'Bhramari Pranayama'. It gets its name from the humming sound you make while practicing it, similar to the sound of a buzzing bee.

Here's how to do it: Close your eyes and take a slow, deep breath in. As you exhale, make a humming sound, like a bee buzzing around a flower. Feel the vibration of the sound in your chest, throat, and head. It's like you're a one-person band, creating music with your breath.

Humming Bee Breath can help calm your mind, reduce anxiety, and even improve your sleep. Plus, it's a great way to add some fun and creativity to your chair yoga practice. Who knew sounding like a bee could be so beneficial?

Cooling Breath

Last on our list is the Cooling Breath or '*Sitali Pranayama*'. This breathing technique is like a natural air conditioner for your body, helping to cool you down and reduce stress.

To practice the Cooling Breath, sit comfortably in your chair. Curl your tongue into a tube shape and stick it out slightly past your lips. Now, take a slow, deep breath in through your mouth, drawing the air over your tongue. Close your mouth and exhale through your nose. Don't worry if you can't roll your tongue. Do your best!

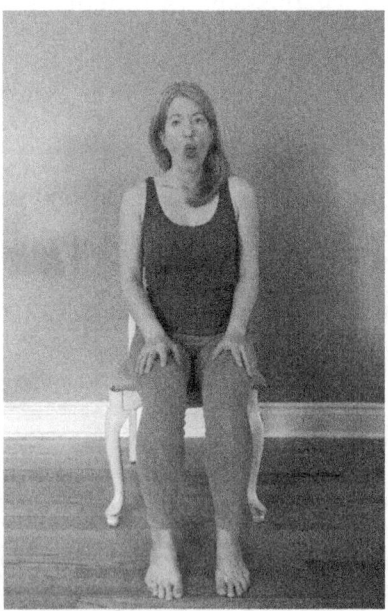

Sitali Pranayama - Cooling breath

Practicing the Cooling Breath during your chair yoga sessions can help lower your body temperature, reduce stress, and promote mental clarity.

To review you now have more breath techniques: diaphragmatic breathing to take you back to your baby days, Humming Bee Breath to add some buzz to your practice, and Cooling Breath to chill out when things heat up. Each of these breathing techniques offers unique benefits and can add a new dimension to your chair yoga practice. So, go on, give them a try, and discover the incredible power of your breath.

Remember, chair yoga is not just about the poses – your breath is an integral part of your practice. It's your rhythm, your guide, and your constant companion through each pose. So, cherish your breath, explore its potential, and let it lead you to new heights in your chair yoga journey. Now, take a deep breath, and let's get ready for the next chapter of our adventure.

CHAPTER FOUR

TAKING SAFETY AND COMFORT TO THE NEXT LEVEL WITH CHAIR YOGA

S itting on a chair, you might be wondering what could possibly go wrong? It's not like you're performing acrobatics on a tightrope. But as with any form of exercise, chair yoga also comes with its own set of guidelines to ensure your safety and enhance your experience. Think of these guidelines as the friendly traffic signals on your chair yoga road trip. They're not there to slow you down, but to ensure you reach your destination safely and enjoyably. So, without further ado, let's explore the golden rules of chair yoga.

The Golden Rules of Chair Yoga

Listen to Your Body

Your body is a lot smarter than you think. It knows when to push harder, when to take a break, and when to call it a day. The key is to tune in and listen to what it's saying.

For instance, if you're doing a seated twist and you feel a sharp pain in your back, that's your body's way of saying, "Hey, this doesn't feel right. Let's stop and try something else." On the other hand, if you feel a gentle stretch in your muscles during a pose, that's your body giving you a thumbs up, encouraging you to keep going.

So, during your chair yoga sessions, make it a point to check in with your body regularly. Pay attention to any sensations, discomfort, or tension, and adjust your movements accordingly. Chair yoga is the perfect practice to learn to tune in to your body's unique needs and responses.

Maintain Proper Alignment

Alignment in yoga is about positioning your body in a way that promotes effectiveness and safety. It's like aligning the wheels of your car for a smoother and safer ride.

In chair yoga, maintaining proper alignment can make a world of difference to your practice. For example, when sitting in your chair, ensure your feet are flat on the floor, your back is straight, and your shoulders are relaxed. This simple alignment can help improve your posture, maximize the benefits of the poses, and reduce the risk of discomfort or injury.

Remember, the goal is not to imitate the pose perfectly, but to find the version of the pose that feels right for you. So, instead of trying to twist like a pretzel, focus on aligning your body in a way that feels comfortable and beneficial.

Don't Forget to Breathe

Breathing is a crucial part of chair yoga. It's like the music that sets the rhythm for your yoga dance. Without it, your practice can feel disjointed and strenuous.

During your chair yoga sessions, make it a point to sync your movements with your breath. Inhale as you stretch or expand your body, and exhale as you fold or contract. This simple act of syncing your breath with your movements can make your practice feel more fluid, focused, and enjoyable.

Remember, your breath is your ally in chair yoga. It guides your movements, helps you stay focused, and even intensifies the benefits of your practice. So, keep breathing, keep moving, and let your breath lead the way.

Now that we're equipped with the golden rules of chair yoga, we're all set to enjoy a safe, effective, and enjoyable practice. But as we progress, keep in mind that these are not rigid rules, but flexible guidelines. They're here to support you, not limit you. So, feel free to adapt them to your needs, listen to your body's wisdom, and most importantly, have fun with your practice. Because at the end of the day, chair yoga is not just about getting fit or losing weight, it's about enjoying the journey, one breath, one pose, one laugh at a time.

How to Avoid Scaring Your Pets While Doing Yoga

You're all set. The comfy chair is in place, your favorite yoga playlist is on, and you're about to enter the zen zone. But wait, what's that furry little obstacle between you and your peaceful practice? Yes, we're talking about your adorable pets who think your yoga time is their playtime. But fret not, dear yogi, because there are simple ways to keep your pets calm and content while you enjoy your chair yoga session. Let's get started!

Choose a Quiet Space

First and foremost, consider the location of your chair yoga practice. The busy, high-traffic living room might not be the wisest choice if you have a curious cat or an energetic dog around and could just invite more interruptions from your pets.

Instead, opt for a quieter, pet-free zone where you can practice in peace. It could be your bedroom, a quiet corner of your study, or even your backyard. The idea is to create a space where you can focus on your practice without any furry distractions.

When my dog was just a puppy, it was nearly impossible for me to practice yoga without her jumping all over me. For some time, I did have to privately close myself in my bedroom. With time, she learned that when I got on my yoga mat, that was my practice and eventually she learned to lay close by while I practiced.

Remember there is no such thing as perfection and the best thing you can do is flow with what is arising.

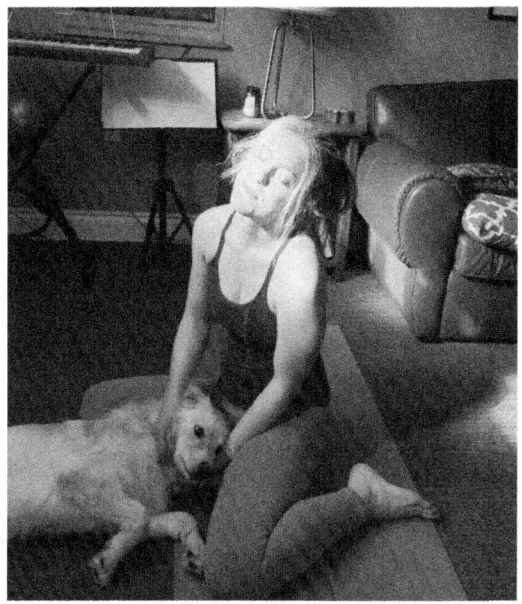

My puppy

Practice Gentle Movements

Finally, consider the nature of your movements during your chair yoga practice. Quick, sudden movements might startle your pets and pique their curiosity. On the other hand, gentle, slow movements are less likely to disturb your pets or disrupt their activities.

Remember, chair yoga is not a race. It's about moving with awareness and grace. So, take your time with each pose, savor each breath, and enjoy the slow, soothing rhythm of your practice. It's like doing a slow dance with your body, keeping your pets calm and your yoga practice uninterrupted.

With a bit of planning and a lot of love for your furry friends, you can enjoy a peaceful chair yoga session, even with your pets around. It's about finding a balance between your fitness goals and the needs of your pets, creating a harmonious environment where everyone can thrive.

So, go ahead, get on comfy, breathable clothes, cue up your playlist, and get ready for a serene chair yoga session. And who knows, your pets might just join in with their own version of Downward Dog or Cat Stretch. Happy practicing!

Chair Yoga: No Band-Aids Required

Warm Up Properly

Just like revving up a car engine on a chilly winter morning, warming up your body before delving into chair yoga is a must-do. It's not about breaking a sweat or flexing those biceps. It's more about waking up your muscles, getting your joints lubricated, and your heart rate slightly elevated.

Imagine you're an actor about to step onto the stage. You wouldn't just walk out and start delivering your lines, would you? Of course not! You'd rehearse, do a couple of voice exercises, and maybe even shake out those nerves. Similarly, warming up before your chair yoga session is about preparing your body and mind for the practice ahead.

So how does one warm up for chair yoga? Start simple. Rotate your ankles, wiggle your toes, roll your shoulders, and turn your head from side to side. Then, maybe do a few gentle twists in your chair, lift your knees one at a time, or stretch your arms overhead. The goal is to get your body moving, shake off that stiffness, and get the blood flowing. You'll be surprised how much smoother your yoga practice will feel after a good warm-up.

Use a Stable Chair

Just as a painter needs a sturdy easel, your chair yoga practice needs a stable chair. It's not about the fancy upholstery or the swiveling feature. It's about having a solid, reliable base for your yoga poses, something that won't wobble or slide around.

Ideally, you want a hard, straight-backed, sturdy chair - something that can withstand your weight and movements without a squeak.

So, what makes a good chair for yoga? Look for something with a flat, firm seat and a straight back. Also, ensure the chair is the right height - your feet should be able to touch the ground comfortably when you're sitting. Armrests can be helpful, but make sure they don't restrict your movements. Remember, your chair is your partner in this chair yoga journey, so choose wisely.

Modify Poses as Needed

Now, here's the thing about chair yoga - it's not a one-size-fits-all kind of deal. It's more like a tailor-made suit, designed to fit you perfectly, with all your unique measurements and quirks. This means you have the freedom, and more importantly, the responsibility, to modify the yoga poses to suit your comfort and ability.

When you go to a restaurant for dinner, you pick and choose what you like, maybe even customize your dish with different sauces or sides. Similarly, in chair yoga, you get to customize your practice. You can modify the poses, change the sequence, or even skip a pose if it doesn't feel right.

The key is to listen to your body and respect its limits. If a pose causes pain or discomfort, it's your body's way of telling you to back off. Don't push through the pain in pursuit of perfection. Instead, find a variant of the pose that feels good and doable. Remember, chair yoga is not about touching your toes; it's about what you learn on the way down. So, embrace the modifications, and make your chair yoga practice your own.

With these safety guidelines in place, you're all set to enjoy chair yoga to the fullest, without risking injuries or discomfort. Remember, chair yoga is a gentle, adaptable practice that's meant to bring you joy, relaxation, and wellness. So, keep these tips in mind, stay safe, and most importantly, enjoy every moment of your chair yoga practice.

Ensuring Your Chair is as Stable as a Mountain

Place the Chair on a Non-Slip Surface

Imagine you're about to go ice skating, but instead of a smooth, icy surface, you're on a sandy beach. It just doesn't work! The same goes for chair yoga. Choosing the right surface for your chair is crucial to ensure a safe and effective practice.

Avoid placing your chair on a slippery or uneven surface, like a polished wooden floor or a thick, plush carpet. Instead, opt for a non-slip mat or a stable, even surface that can provide a firm grip for your chair.

Think of it this way: you're creating a sturdy foundation for your chair yoga practice, just like the roots of a tree anchoring it firmly to the ground. This way, you can focus on your poses without worrying about your chair slipping or sliding around.

Use a Chair with Arms for Extra Support

Now, let's talk about the chair itself. Not all chairs are created equal, especially when it comes to chair yoga. The star of the show here is a chair with arms.

The arms of a chair serve a similar purpose during your yoga practice. They provide extra support and stability, especially during challenging poses or transitions.

The armrests act as your personal spotter, ready to lend a helping hand whenever you need it. So, whether you're twisting, stretching, or balancing, you can lean on these trusty armrests for added support and stability.

Avoid Overstretching or Leaning Too Far

Last but not least, let's talk about the poses themselves. The beauty of chair yoga lies in its adaptability. You can modify the poses to suit your comfort level, ensuring a safe and enjoyable practice.

But here's the catch: while it's tempting to stretch a little further or twist a little deeper, it's important not to overdo it. Overstretching or leaning too far can put strain on your muscles and joints, and may even tip your chair.

Listen to your body's cues and respect its limits. If a pose causes discomfort or feels unstable, ease out of it and try a gentler version.

Remember, chair yoga is not about touching your toes or twisting like a pretzel. It's about finding a balance between effort and ease, challenge and comfort, movement and stillness. So, take it slow, keep it safe, and most importantly, enjoy the ride.

And that, dear reader, wraps up our guide to a safe and comfortable chair yoga practice. So, the next time you settle into your chair for a yoga session, remember these guidelines. They're your roadmap to a safe, effective, and enjoyable practice. Remember, your chair is not just a piece of furniture; it's your partner on this exciting fitness adventure. So, treat it with care, respect its role, and together, you'll create a chair yoga symphony that's harmonious, uplifting, and uniquely yours. As we move on, we'll explore the diverse world of chair yoga poses, adding new notes to our symphony. So, stay tuned, keep practicing, and let's continue this incredible journey together.

CHAPTER FIVE

HOW YOUR CHAIR CAN HELP YOU SHED POUNDS

You're sitting comfortably in your favorite chair, feet firmly on the floor, and a smile on your face. It seems like the perfect setting for a relaxing evening, doesn't it? But what if I told you that this very chair could be your secret weapon in your battle against the bulge? Don't believe me? Stick around, because we're about to uncover the surprising weight-loss potential of chair yoga. Skeptics- hold onto your armrests. This is going to be an eye-opener!

How Chair Yoga Helps Melt Pounds

Calorie Burning Poses

Let's cut to the chase. Can sitting on a chair really burn calories? The answer is a resounding yes! Each pose in chair yoga involves movement and muscle engagement, which means your body is burning calories.

Consider the seated mountain pose, for instance. As simple as it may seem, this pose engages your core, strengthens your spine, and improves your posture. It's like doing a mini workout for your midsection, all while sitting down. And the best part? You're burning calories without even breaking a sweat!

Metabolism Boosting Techniques

Now, burning calories is one side of the weight loss coin. The other side is your metabolism, the rate at which your body burns calories. The faster your metabolism, the more calories you burn, even when you're at rest. And here's the kicker: chair yoga can help boost your metabolism!

When you practice chair yoga regularly, you're not just burning calories; you're also building lean muscle mass. And guess what? Muscle burns more calories than fat, even when you're at rest. So, the more muscle you have, the higher your resting metabolic rate.

Fat Burning Breathing Exercises

Wait a minute, can breathing really burn fat? It sounds far-fetched, but the truth is, that breathing exercises, or *pranayama*, can play a crucial role in weight loss.

Breathing deeply increases the amount of oxygen in your body. This oxygen is needed to burn fat for energy. So, the more oxygen you have, the more fat you can potentially burn.

When you stoke a campfire to keep it burning brightly, the more air you fan into the fire, the brighter it burns. Similarly, the deeper you breathe, the more oxygen you fan into your body's metabolic fire, helping it burn fat more effectively.

Take the '*breath of fire*', for instance. This breathing technique involves rapid, forceful breaths that increase the flow of oxygen in your body, ramp up your metabolic rate, and help burn fat. It's an incredibly detoxifying breath. I go into more detail about the breath of fire in Chapter 8 with energizing breathwork.

Chair yoga isn't just about stretching and strengthening; it's also about burning calories, boosting metabolism, and even burning fat through breathing exercises. It's a holistic, three-pronged approach to weight loss that doesn't require heavy weights, fancy equipment, or even standing up. All you need is a chair, your body, and the willingness to try something new. So, are you ready to turn your chair into a calorie-burning, fat-blasting, metabolism-boosting machine? Let's do this!

The Surprise Element of Chair Yoga for Weight Loss

Unexpected Muscle Engagement

So you are all set up sitting on your chair, ready to dive into a chair yoga session. As you sit there, you might be thinking, "How many muscles could I possibly engage while seated?" Well, prepare to be pleasantly surprised!

Consider the Seated Mountain Pose. As you sit upright, feet flat on the floor, hands resting on your thighs, you're not just sitting. You're actively engaging your core muscles, strengthening your spine, and even working those leg muscles. It's like having an undercover gym session while sitting in your chair!

Now, let's say you move into a Chair Hip Stretch, where you cross one ankle over the opposite knee and gently press down on the raised knee. You're not just stretching your hip muscles; you're also engaging your core, your glutes, and even your back muscles.

Don't worry! Both of those poses mentioned will be taught in detail in the next chapter.

So, as you can see, chair yoga is not just about gentle stretches or deep breaths. It's a full-body workout that engages various muscle groups, often in ways you wouldn't expect. And the best part? You're toning and strengthening your muscles without even leaving your chair!

Hidden Cardiovascular Benefits

Now, let's talk about your heart. No, not the one that skips a beat when you see your favorite dessert, but the one that works tirelessly to keep you alive and kicking. You might be wondering, "Can chair yoga really benefit my heart?" The answer is a resounding yes!

You see, each time you move your body, stretch your muscles, or take a deep breath, you're making your heart work a bit harder. It's like taking your heart on a gentle jog, increasing its rate, and pumping more blood throughout your body. This increased heart rate can help improve your cardiovascular fitness, even though you're not huffing and puffing or sweating buckets.

Moreover, the deep, mindful breathing practices in chair yoga can help lower your blood pressure and reduce stress, both of which are excellent for heart health. It's like giving your heart a soothing massage, helping it relax and function more efficiently.

So yes, chair yoga does have hidden cardiovascular benefits!

Unseen Flexibility Improvements

Remember those days when touching your toes seemed as impossible as climbing Mount Everest? Well, prepare to be amazed, because chair yoga can significantly improve your flexibility, often in ways you wouldn't expect.

Take the Seated Forward Bend, for instance. As you hinge forward from your hips, reaching for your toes, you're not just giving your back a good stretch. You're also increasing the flexibility of your hamstrings, your spine, and even your neck muscles.

Now, you probably will not become super flexible overnight... But with regular practice, you'll notice improvements in your flexibility. You might find it easier to reach for that top shelf or bend down to tie your shoelaces or twist around to reverse your car. It's the unseen flexibility improvements that make chair yoga such a game-changer.

Chair yoga is full of surprises. It's not just about sitting and stretching; it's about engaging muscles you never knew you had, giving your heart a gentle workout, and becoming more flexible in ways you didn't think possible. All this, without even standing up!

Are you ready to unlock the surprises of chair yoga? Your chair is waiting, and so is your healthier, fitter, and more flexible self! Let's get moving.

Your Chair: The Secret to Fitting into Those Old Jeans

Waistline Focused Poses

Alright, let's talk about waistlines. Now, I'm not here to preach about the "perfect" waist size or make you feel guilty about that extra slice of pizza you enjoyed last night. Instead, let's discover how chair yoga can support a healthier waistline, and yes, help you slip into those snug jeans hiding at the back of your closet.

Let's start with the Seated Twist. Picture yourself sitting tall and proud in your chair, feet flat on the floor. Now, imagine you're in the middle of a thrilling mystery novel, and there's a sudden plot twist. You'd turn the pages eagerly, right? In the Seated Twist, you turn your body instead. As you rotate your upper body to one side, keeping your hips and legs stable, you're giving your waist a gentle, yet effective workout. It's like wringing out a wet towel, only you're wringing out tension from your body and toning your waistline at the same time.

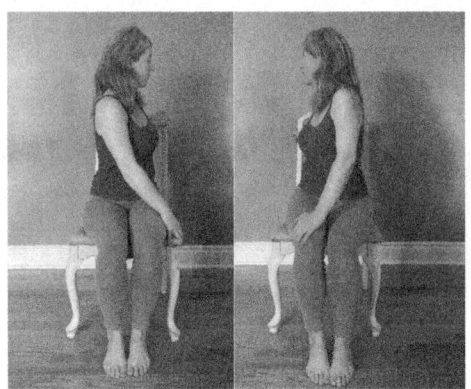

Seated Twist

Abdominal Strengthening Techniques

Now let's shift our focus a bit lower to the powerhouse of your body - your abs. You might be thinking, "Can I really work on my abs while sitting?" To that, I say, bring on the Seated Boat Pose!

Imagine you're on a boat, gently rocking on a calm lake. Now, let's bring that boat onto your chair. Sit a bit forward on your chair so that there is some space between your back and the back of the chair, lean back slightly, and lift your legs off the floor. Breathe deeply and hold for as long as you can. Feel your abs working to keep you balanced? That's your seated boat, toning your abs without a single sit-up or crunch.

This is a challenging pose on and off the chair! Lower your legs closer to the ground to make it a bit easier. Alternatively, you can keep your feet flat on the floor. Lean your upper body back in a straight line on an angle. Arms are alongside your body. Engage your core muscles.

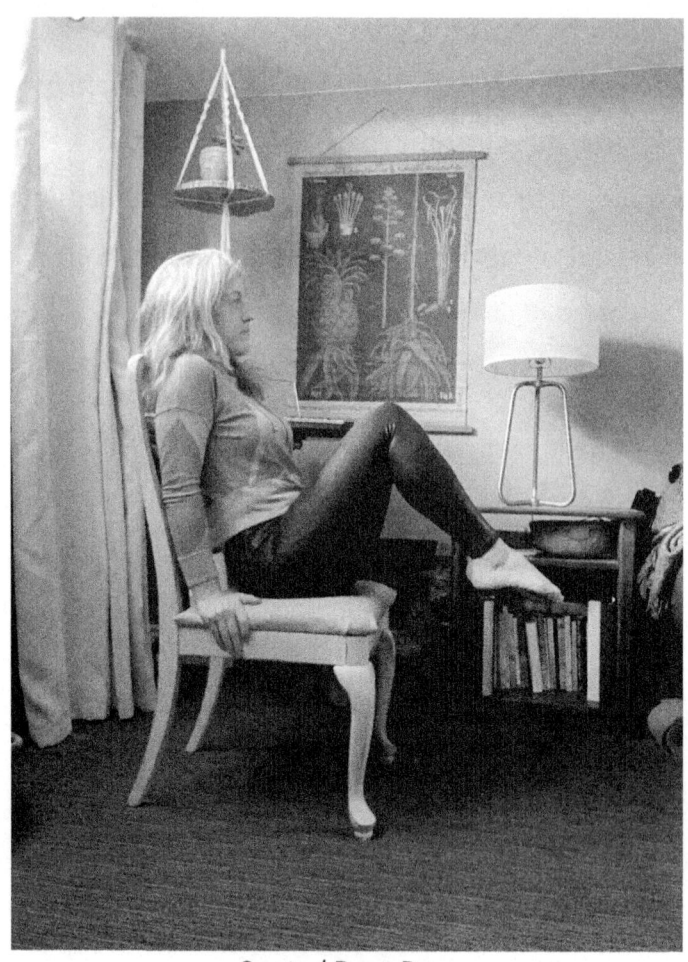

Seated Boat Pose

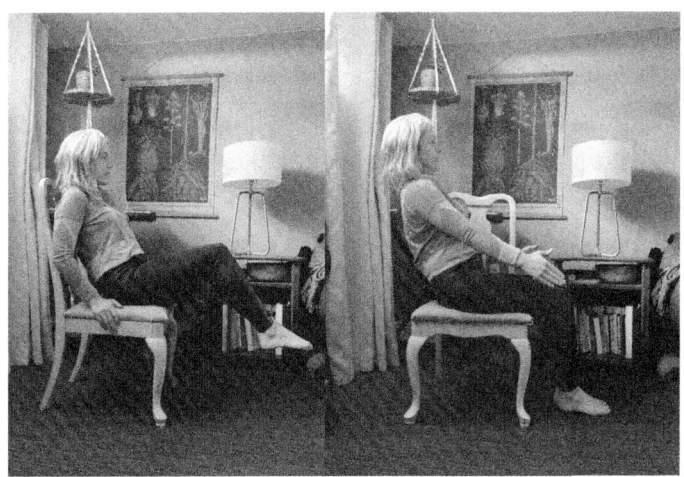

Variation I for Seated Boat Pose: Lowering legs closer to ground.

Variation II for Seated Boat Pose: Feet flat on floor. Leaning back slightly. Engaging Core.

Hip and Thigh Slimming Exercises

Okay, let's move further down to your hips and thighs. Yes, we're going to target those stubborn areas with some chair yoga magic. Enter the Supported Bridge Pose.

Think about a beautiful bridge arching over a serene river. Now let's build that bridge in your chair.

Seated Bridge pose does involve coming onto the ground and using the chair for support. If this is not something accessible for you, skip this pose.

You come lying down in front of your chair. You elevate your lower legs on the seat of the chair and breathe deeply.

To kick it up a notch and if you feel like a challenge, bring your feet flat on the seat of the chair. Then, push down on your feet, lifting your hips and thighs into the air. Breathe deeply while you hold here. Can you feel those muscles working? Congratulations! You've just built a bridge to slimmer hips and thighs.

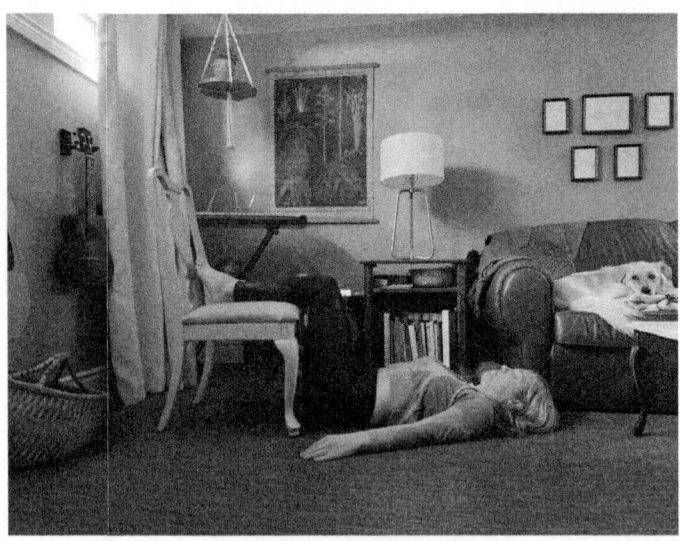

Supported Bridge Pose

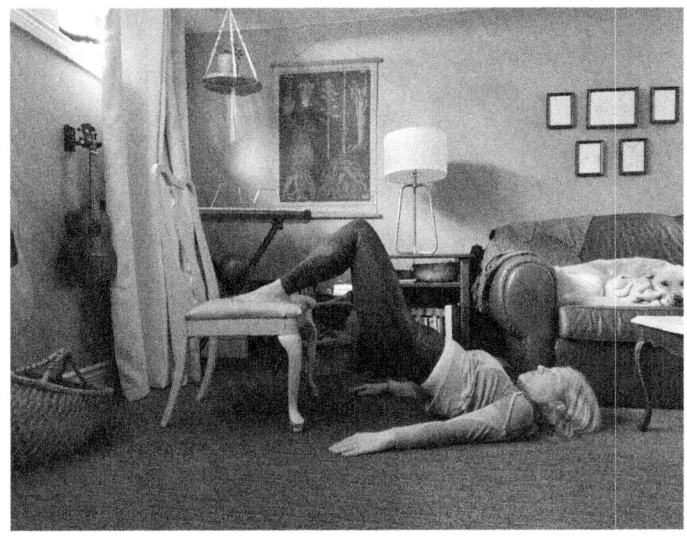

Lifted Bridge

Chair yoga isn't just about stretching and relaxing; it's about building strength, toning muscles, and yes, helping you fit into your favorite jeans. And the best part? You're doing all this while sitting down. No huffing and puffing, no fancy gym equipment, and definitely no guilt trips. Just you, your chair, and a healthier, happier body. Now, that's what I call a win-win!

So, go ahead, and give these poses a try. Embrace the twists, rock the boat, and build that bridge. Your body will thank you for it, and who knows, those old jeans might just make a comeback! Enjoy your practice, celebrate your progress, and remember, you're not just doing yoga; you're creating a healthier, happier, more mobile you.

Let's keep the momentum going. Up next, we'll uncover more chair yoga poses that are not just fun and relaxing, but also incredibly effective for weight loss. We'll delve even deeper into the world of poses, breathing techniques, and the nitty-gritty of a successful chair yoga routine. So, stay tuned, keep practicing, and let's continue to unlock the amazing potential of chair yoga.

Your body will thank you for it!

CHAPTER SIX

GET MOVING, KEEP SMILING

CHAIR YOGA FUNDAMENTALS

The chair yoga poses in this chapter will be a solid foundation to make you stronger, more flexible, and significantly lighter (on the scale and in spirit)! It's packed with simple, fun, and effective chair yoga poses designed especially for beginners and seniors. Something I suggest to my clients is this: If you're spending a large amount of time sitting in your living room watching TV or binging on Netflix - why not engage your body and get some stretching and exercise as well! Intrigued? Let's get started.

Chair Yoga Poses That Won't Make You Sweat Profusely

Chair Cat-Cow Stretch

Have you ever watched a cat stretch after a long nap? There's something incredibly graceful and satisfying about it. The Chair Cat-Cow Stretch draws inspiration from our feline friends, helping to stretch and strengthen your spine.

Here's how to do it:

- Sit up tall on your chair, feet flat on the floor.

- Place your hands on your knees.

- As you inhale, arch your back and stick your chest forward. Look up towards the ceiling (this is the Cow part).

- As you exhale, round your back and drop your head towards your chest (this is the Cat part).

- Repeat this sequence a few times, moving with your breath. Breathe deeply!

- Pro tip: Try this pose in the morning to wake up your spine and start your day on a positive note.

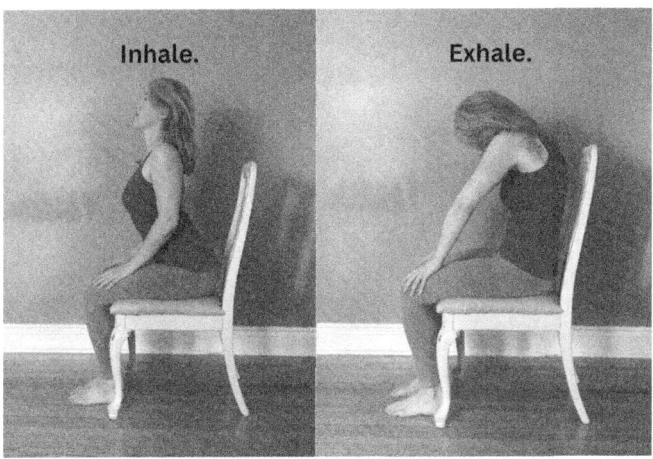

Inhale. Exhale.

Seated Cat and Cow

Chair Sufi Grinding

I love this warm-up exercise that wakes up your entire spine and gives your internal organs a beautiful massage. I teach it as a warm-up in all of my classes and with my private clients. My clients call this exercise "feels like heaven." The best part is anyone can do it and it most definitely can be done every day as a spinal tune-up and a way to give yourself some love.

Here's how to do it:

- Sit up tall on your chair, feet flat on the floor.

- Place your hands on your thighs.

- As you inhale, you rotate your torso to the front in a circle as you arch your back and stick your chest out.

- As you exhale, you rotate your torso in a circular motion toward the back as you round your back.

- You are rotating your torso in a circular motion over the top of your pelvis.

- Think of this motion as a mortar and pestle grinding spices. Your torso grinds down into the bowl (your pelvic bowl) as it is rotating in circles.

- Repeat this sequence a few times, moving with your breath in one direction. Then move in circles the other way. Breathe deeply!

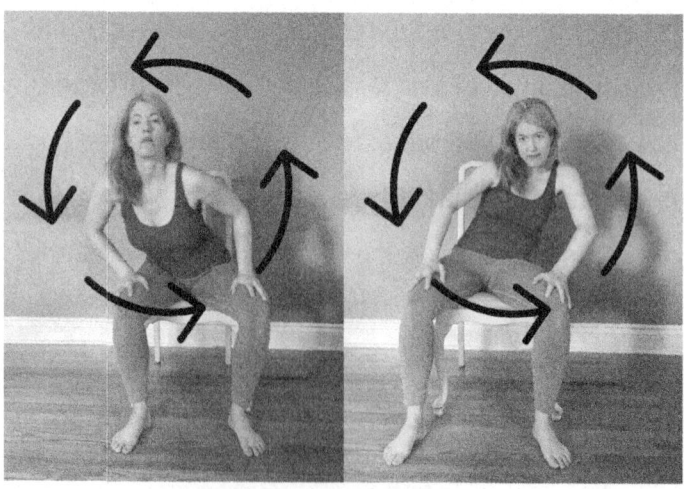

Chair Sufi Grinding

Chair Raised Hands Pose

Let's move on to the Chair Raised Hands Pose, a simple yet powerful pose that stretches your entire body.

Here's how to do it:

- Sit up tall on your chair, feet flat on the floor.

- As you inhale, raise your arms overhead, reaching towards the ceiling.

- Keep your shoulders relaxed and away from your ears.

- Hold for a few breaths, then release your arms back down as you exhale.

- Pro tip: Use this pose as a quick pick-me-up during your midday slump. It's even more refreshing than a cup of coffee!

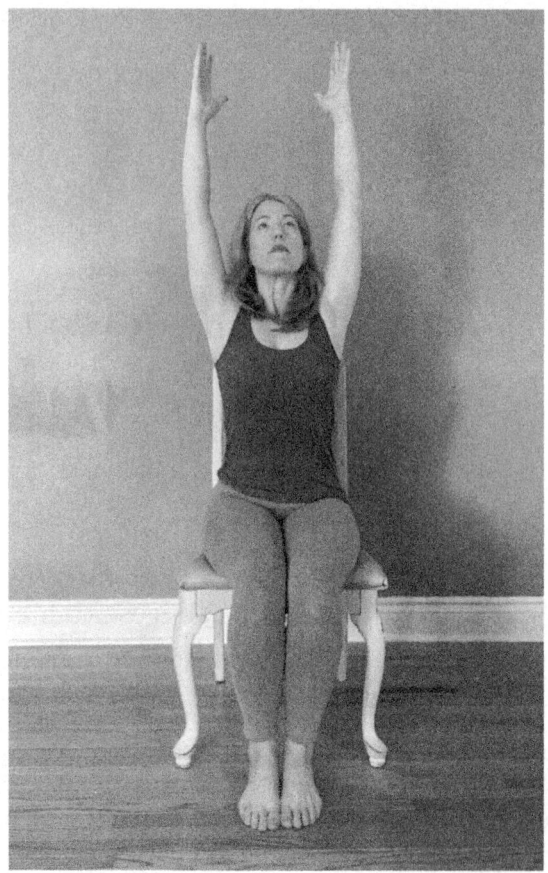

Chair Raised Hands Pose

Chair Neck Turns

This is a gentle way to release tension in your neck.

Here's how to do it:

- Sit up tall on your chair, feet flat on the floor.

- Inhale and slowly turn your head to the left.

- Exhale and slowly turn your head to the right.

- It seems simple, but the slow intention and syncing with your breath brings mindfulness to this and has great benefit.

- This simple exercise is great for your thyroid as well!

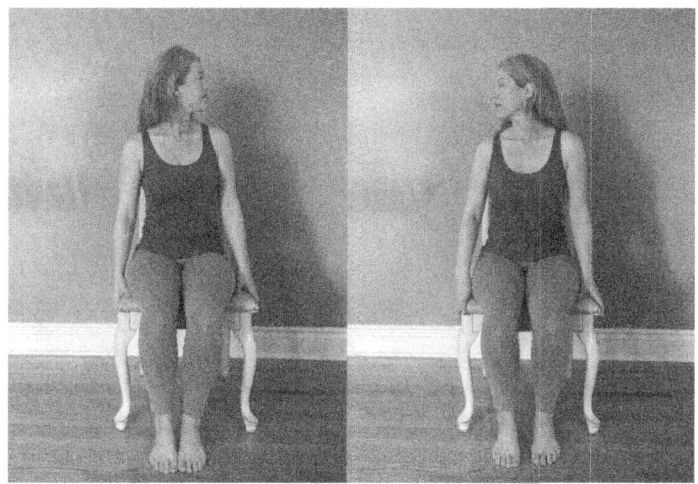

Neck Turns

Chair Forward Bend

Next up, we have the Chair Forward Bend. It's like giving your body a big, loving hug.

Here's how to do it:

- Sit on your chair, feet flat on the floor.

- Take a deep breath in, and as you exhale, fold forward from your hips, letting your torso rest on your thighs.

- Let your head hang down towards your knees, and relax your arms on the floor.

- Stay in this pose for a few deep breaths, then slowly roll up to sitting as you inhale.

- Pro tip: Try this pose at the end of a long day to release tension and stress from your body.

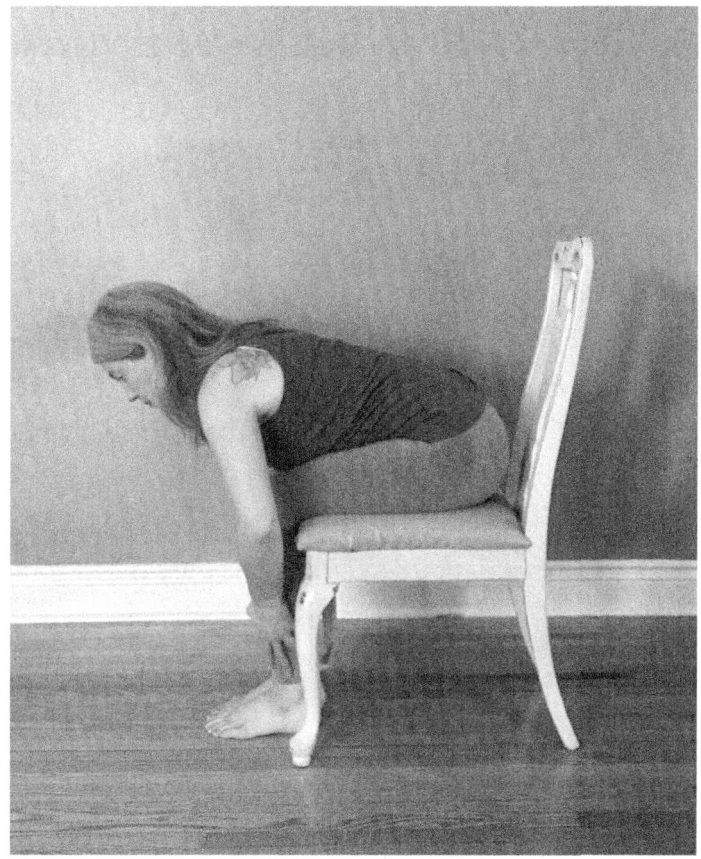

Chair Forward Bend

There you have it, five simple chair yoga poses that won't make you sweat profusely but will get your body moving and your spirits lifting. Remember, the goal here is not to become a chair yoga master overnight. It's about exploring your body's capabilities, enjoying the process, and most importantly, having fun! Up next, we have some poses that you can even do while watching TV. Sounds exciting? Let's keep going!

Simple Poses That Can Be Done While Watching TV

Chair Mountain Pose

Tuning into your favorite TV show? Great! But let's not forget our body in the process. The Chair Mountain Pose is a perfect starting point. It's like being the star of your own show, right there in your living room.

To get into the pose, sit up as straight as possible in your chair. Plant your feet flat on the floor, hip-width apart. Keep your back straight, shoulders down relaxed, and hands resting gently on your thighs. Imagine yourself as a majestic mountain, grounded yet reaching for the sky. Hold this pose for a few breaths, feeling your body aligning with your breath.

The beauty of the Chair Mountain Pose is its subtlety. It may not look like much, but it's working wonders on your posture, core strength, and mental focus. It's definitely a different way to engage your body beneficially while you're tuning into your favorite Netflix series. The best part is it starts to bring awareness to your posture so that this can start to ripple out into your way of moving, sitting, and standing all the time.

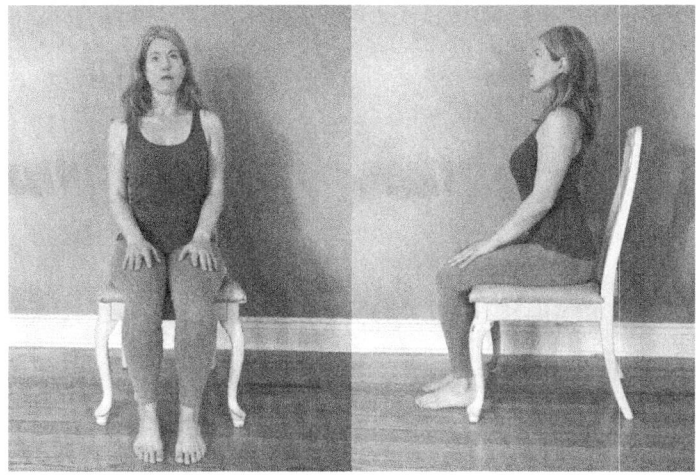

Chair Mountain Pose

Chair Eagle Pose

Next up, let's weave in the Chair Eagle Pose. Picture yourself as a mighty eagle soaring high above the clouds. Ready to take flight?

Start in your Mountain Pose, sit up straight, and extend your arms out in front of you. Cross your right arm over the left, bending at the elbows. If possible, twist your forearms around each other, pressing your palms together. Next, cross your right thigh over the left, hooking your right foot behind the left calf if it feels comfortable. If this does not work for your body, keep your feet flat on the ground.

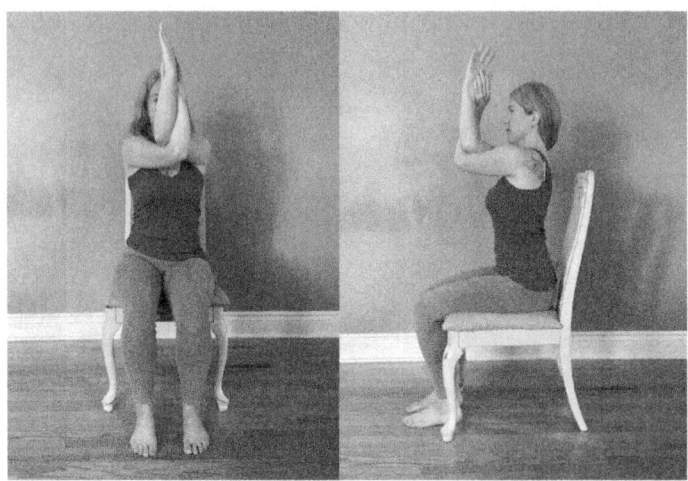

Chair Eagle Pose

If you can't twist your arms like that - it's okay! An alternative is to give yourself a big hug! Stack your arms so the left is under the right and grab the backs of your shoulders. Also, be mindful to gently pull your shoulders down and forward.

This will ensure you get a lovely stretch in your upper back, specifically in the scapula and trapezius region where many of us hold so much tension.

Hold the pose for a few breaths, feeling the stretch in your shoulders, arms, and legs. Unwind slowly and repeat on the other side.

On the other side - you are simply switching your arms so that your left arm crosses over your right. Next, cross your left thigh over your right.

The Chair Eagle Pose is like a mini adventure during your downtime, offering a full-body stretch and a dash of fun.

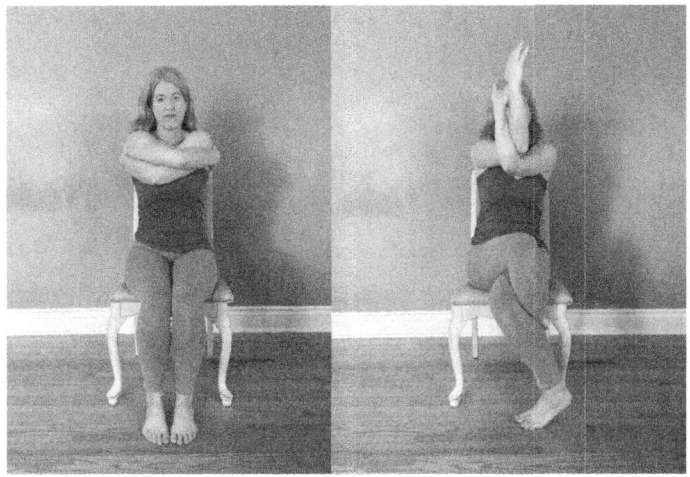

Variations for Chair Eagle Pose

Chair Warrior I Pose

Now, let's add some drama to our prime-time attraction with the Chair Warrior I Pose. Imagine yourself as a warrior, strong, brave, and ready for action. You get to be your own superhero, standing tall and confident, ready to take on the world. Sounds exciting, right? Let's bring that excitement to your chair!

To get into the pose, sit sideways on your chair, one leg bent at the knee and the other extended straight out behind you. Reach your arms overhead, palms facing each other. Lift your chest, pull your shoulders back, and look up towards your hands. Turn your upper body to face forward, keeping your hips aligned.

Hold the pose for a few breaths, feeling the stretch in your chest, arms, and legs. Slowly release and repeat on the other side. The Chair Warrior I Pose is like a power-packed scene in your favorite action movie. It's exciting, energizing, and keeps you on the edge of your seat, quite literally! This pose works your core and leg muscles, increasing your flexibility, and boosting your mood. Who knew your chair could be this much fun?

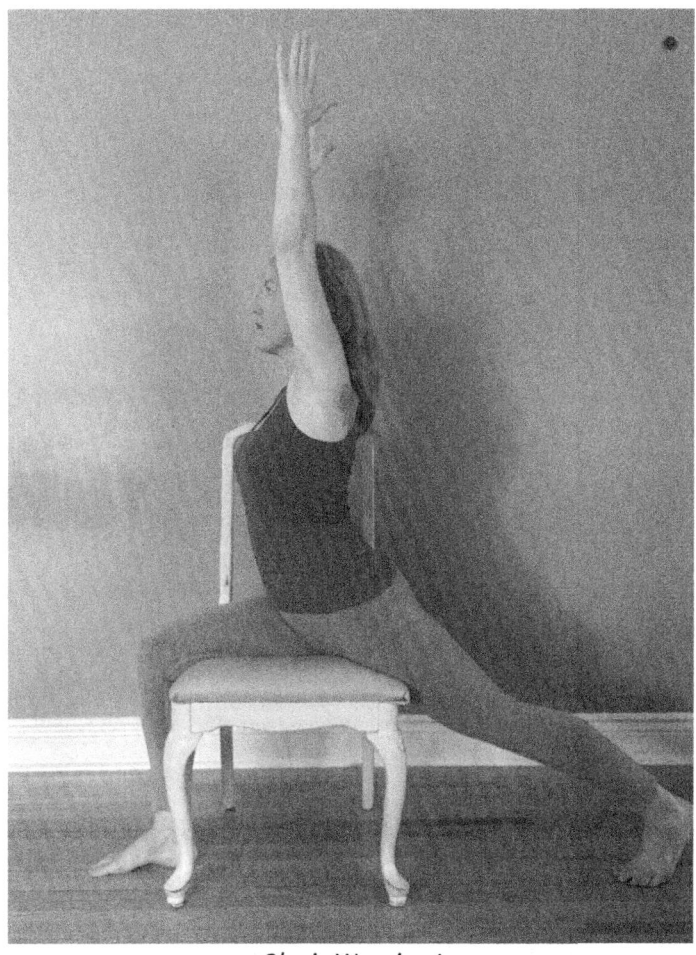

Chair Warrior I

You have just learned three simple chair yoga poses that you can do while watching TV. These poses bring a dash of movement, a sprinkle of fun, and a whole lot of health benefits to your viewing time. They're easy, effective, and can be done without missing a beat of your favorite show. So, why wait? Grab your remote, tune into your favorite channel, and let's get moving with chair yoga - the ultimate way to maximize your downtime and feel good!

Yoga Poses That Your Cat Can't Do

Chair Spinal Twist

Next up, we have the Chair Twist, a pose that's all about rotation and rejuvenation.

While seated, place your right hand on your left knee and your left hand on the backrest of your chair. As you inhale, sit up tall, and as you exhale, gently twist your upper body to the left. Hold the pose for a few breaths, then slowly untwist and repeat on the other side.

The Chair Twist is like a mini detox for your body, wringing out tension and refreshing your spine. It's a gentle, yet effective way to add some movement and flexibility to your chair yoga practice.

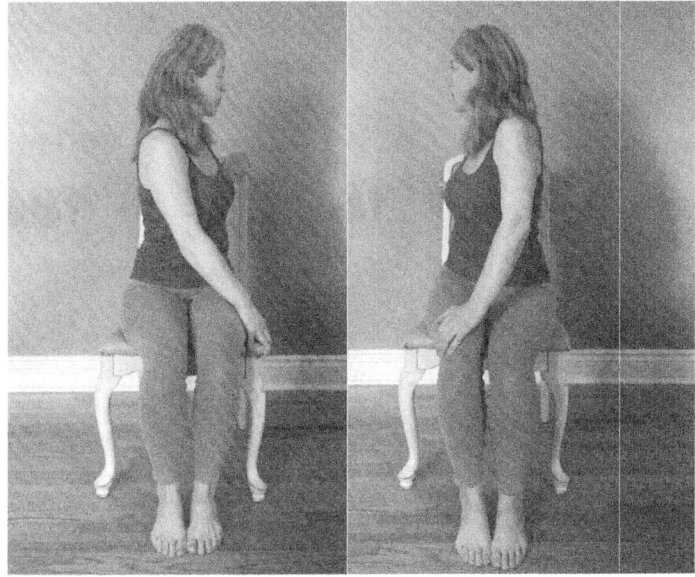

Chair Spinal Twist

Chair Hip Stretch

Finally, let's explore the Chair Hip Stretch, a pose that's sure to make your hips happy. When you reach for a high shelf in your kitchen, the stretch you're emulating is essentially the Chair Hip Stretch.

Here's how you do it: Sit up straight on your chair, feet flat on the floor. Cross your right ankle over your left knee, creating a figure '4' with your legs. Rest your right hand on your right knee and gently press down, feeling a stretch in your right hip. Hold the pose for a few breaths, then gently release and repeat on the other side.

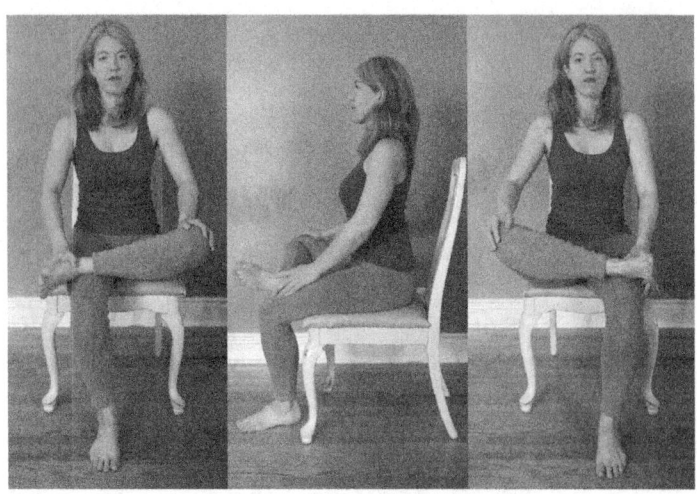

Chair Hip Stretch

The Chair Hip Stretch is like a soothing massage for your hips, releasing tension and increasing flexibility. It's a simple, yet powerful way to add some spice to your chair yoga routine. If you have lower back pain or struggle with sciatica pain, this pose is one to practice every day. Plus, it's a pose that even your cat can't do!

So we covered two unique chair yoga poses that are fun, effective, and definitely not boring. They're your secret weapons in your journey towards better health, greater flexibility, and a happier you. So, get cozy in your chair, try these poses, and discover the magic of chair yoga. Your body will thank you for it, and who knows, you might just find yourself looking forward to your chair yoga sessions more than your favorite TV show. Now, wouldn't that be something?

Calorie-Burning Poses: Easy and Effective

Chair Sun Salutation: Greet the Day with Energy

The Sun Salutation, or Surya Namaskar, is a series of twelve poses performed in a flow in traditional yoga. The adapted version for chair yoga keeps the essence and flow of the original sequence intact, making it an accessible and invigorating practice right from your chair.

As you start your Chair Sun Salutation, imagine that you are there to greet the day with energy and vitality. Begin in a seated mountain pose, with your hands at the heart center. As you breathe in, sweep your arms up overhead, arching your back slightly into a gentle backbend to welcome the day.

On your next exhale, fold forward over your legs into a forward bend, letting your hands rest on your shins or the floor. Then, as you inhale, lift your torso halfway, extending your spine and looking forward, like a halfway lift in traditional yoga.

Exhale and fold forward once again, before inhaling as you sweep your arms out to the sides and overhead, coming back to the gentle backbend. Finally, as you exhale, bring your hands back to the heart center (or your sternum).

The idea is that you repeat this sequence a few times at your own pace in rhythm with your breath. This is the Vinyasa flow discussed earlier. It's like a yoga dance but you get to determine the pace, the energy you bring to it, and how gracefully you move through it.

The Chair Sun Salutation is a calorie-burning powerhouse, engaging multiple muscle groups in one fluid sequence, and getting your heart rate up. It's like weaving a beautiful tapestry of poses, each thread contributing to a vibrant picture of vitality and health.

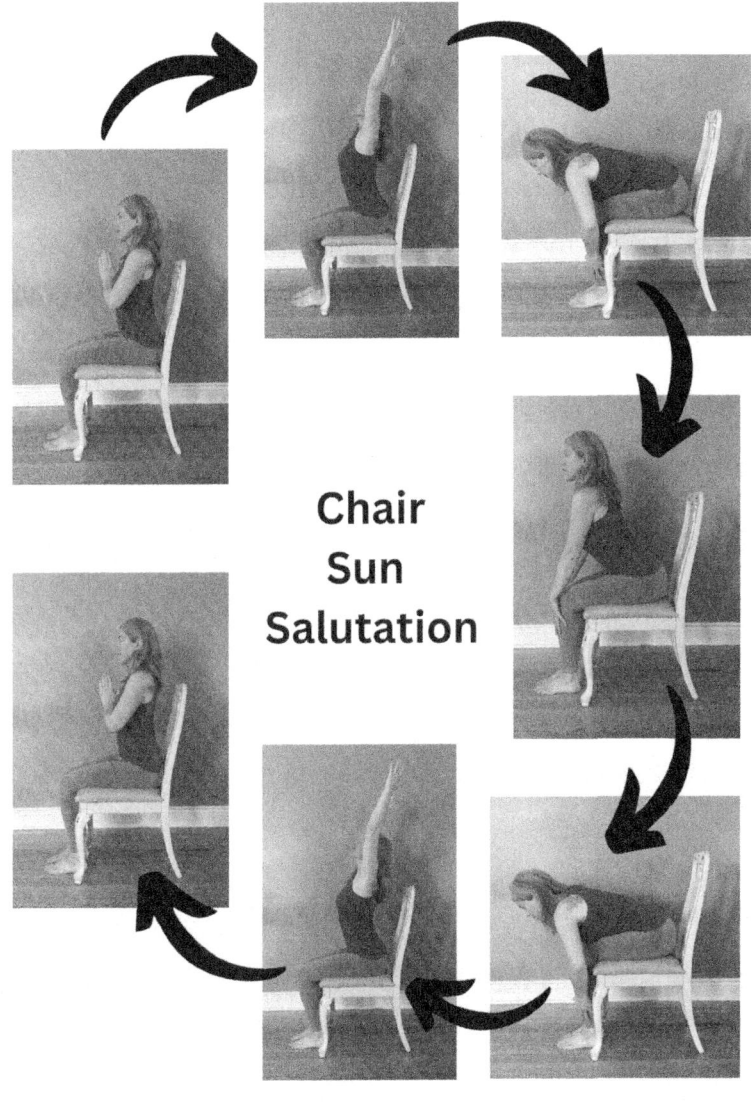

Chair
Sun
Salutation

Chair Savasana: The Art of Conscious Relaxation

Now, let's shift gears and explore the most relaxed pose in yoga – Savasana, or Corpse Pose. Don't let the name scare you off. In chair yoga, Savasana is all about conscious relaxation, where you give your body permission to rest and absorb the benefits of your practice. This pose may be most comfortable on a big soft armchair as opposed to a straightback chair. This is because you are really giving your weight into the chair so you want to be comfortable.

Imagine you're a cloud floating in a clear blue sky. Nothing to do, nowhere to go. Just being. That's the essence of Chair Savasana. Sit back in your chair, let your hands rest comfortably on your thighs or by your sides, and close your eyes. Let your body sink into the chair, and bring your attention to your breath.

As you rest in Chair Savasana, your body switches into the rest-and-digest mode, where it starts repairing tissues, strengthening the immune system, and yes, burning calories. It's like your body's maintenance crew getting to work, ensuring everything is running smoothly.

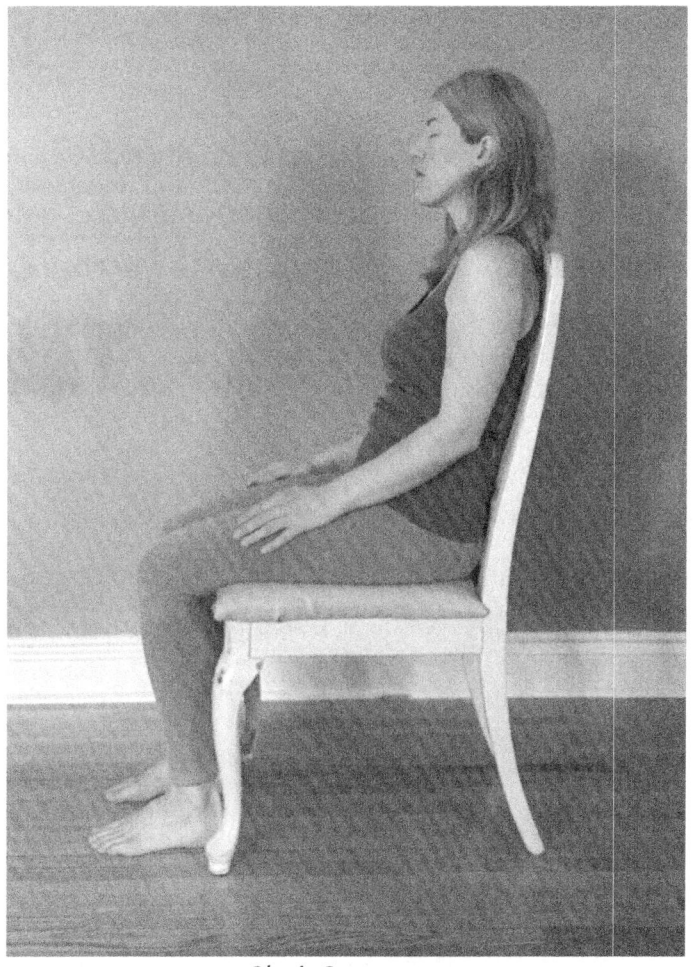

Chair Savasana

Chair Tree Pose: Balance, Strength, and Calm

Last but not least, let's venture into the forest with the Chair
Tree Pose. Just like a tall, sturdy tree, roots reaching deep
into the earth, branches reaching high into the sky - you

get to become strong and sturdy and root down. That's the image we'll embody in Chair Tree Pose.

To get into the pose, start in a seated mountain pose. Then, shift your weight onto your right buttock and place your left foot on the inside of your right leg, either above or below the knee. Just don't rest your foot directly on your knee! You can also place a yoga block on the floor and use that to place your foot on. This is a gentle variation.

Press your left knee gently towards the left side, opening the hip. Bring your hands to the heart center, and voila, you're a tree! Keep breathing deeply as this will help your focus and your balance.

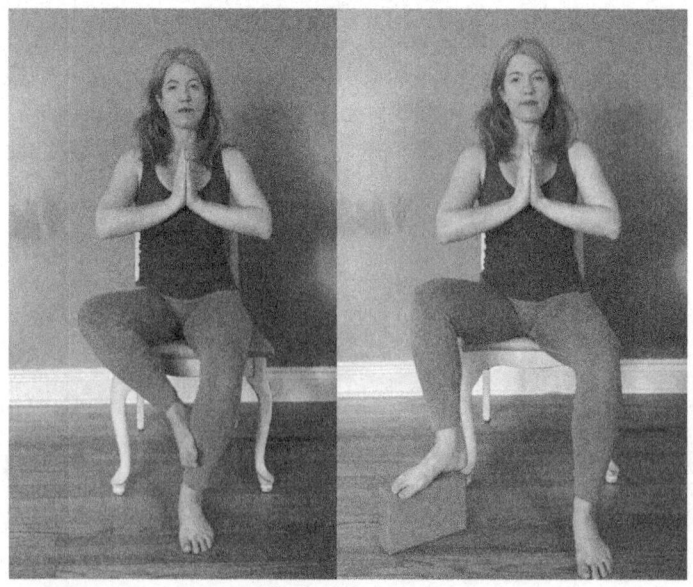

Chair Tree Pose

The Chair Tree Pose is not just about balance and strength; it's also about inner calm. As you hold the pose, your body is burning calories, your mind is focused, and you're cultivating a sense of peace and stability. It's like you're a tree, weathering the storms with grace and resilience.

When you feel ready you can come standing and use your chair to help balance. From a fully standing position, hold onto the back of your chair with your right hand. Lift that left foot on the inside of your right leg. Remember not to rest your foot on your knee! Push that left knee out and open up the hip. Bring your left arm up high above your head and tall like a tree. Hold and breathe deeply. Then, repeat on the other leg.

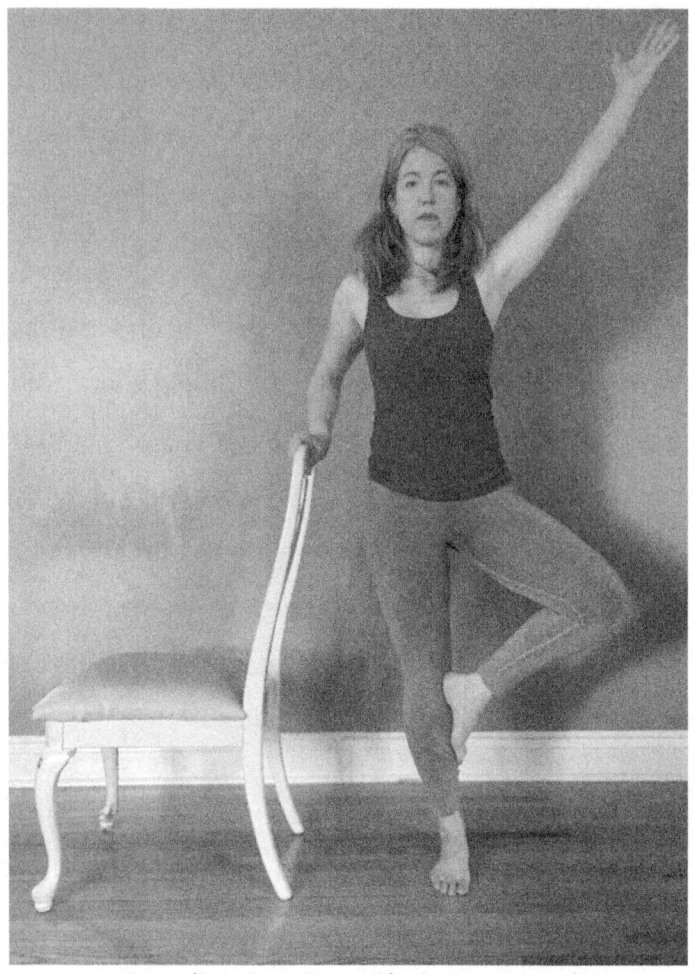

Standing Tree Pose Chair-Supported

You now have a full sequence with the Sun Salutation where you can find your own flow. The last two yoga poses are effective chair yoga poses that can help burn calories and enhance your overall fitness. They're your secret weapons in your quest for weight loss, right there in your chair. So, go ahead, greet the sun, rest like a cloud, and stand tall like a tree. Your chair yoga adventure is just getting started!

As we continue to explore the fascinating world of chair yoga, keep these poses in your toolkit. They're not just exercises; they're stepping stones to a healthier, happier you. Remember, every breath counts, every pose matters, and every moment on your chair brings you closer to your wellness goals. So, keep practicing, keep exploring, and most importantly, keep having fun with chair yoga. Your journey to wellness is well on its way.

Up next, we'll delve deeper into the world of chair yoga, uncovering more poses, more tips, and more surprises. So, stay tuned, and let's keep the momentum going. Your chair is waiting, and so is your journey to a healthier, happier you.

CHAPTER SEVEN

DISCOVERING YOUR INNER STRENGTH

THE JOY OF PELVIC FLOOR YOGA

Alright, let's play a quick game of word association. I say "yoga", you say... "pelvic floor"? Wait, what? Yes, you heard it right. We're about to dive into the world of pelvic floor yoga - a somewhat overlooked, but incredibly beneficial aspect of yoga and one that I am particularly passionate about.

The Power of the Pelvic Floor: More than Just Muscle

Understanding the Pelvic Floor

Think of your body as a bustling city, and your pelvic floor as the intricate subway system underneath. It's a complex network of muscles that forms the base of your pelvis, connecting various parts of your body, much like subway lines connect different parts of the city.

This network of muscles plays a crucial role in maintaining bladder and bowel control, and sexual function. They're like the unsung heroes of your body, working quietly in the background, ensuring everything runs smoothly.

Pelvic floor exercises involve contracting and relaxing the pelvic floor muscles, which can be done while seated, making them accessible for seniors and beginners to chair yoga.

Female Pelvic Floor Muscles

Public Crest	Public Sumphysis
Urethral Canal	Bulb Of Vestibule
Vaginal Canal	Posterior Fourchette
Pubococcygeus	
Rectal Canal	External Anal Sphinster Muscle
Iliococcygeus	Perineal Body
Iliacus	Levator Ani Muscle
Sacrum	Iliac Crests

The Pelvic Floor and Incontinence

According to the Continence Foundation of Australia, strong pelvic floor muscles are essential for preventing and managing urinary incontinence, particularly in the senior population. Engaging in pelvic floor exercises while sitting on a chair is a non-surgical way of dealing with incontinence. When chair-based pelvic floor yoga can be incorporated into your daily routine, over time, this daily habit will lead to noticeable improvements.

Noticeable Improvements Over Time

I can't get this point across enough! With any yoga practice, including pelvic floor yoga, regular practice is key! Just like a seed gradually grows into a mighty tree, the benefits of pelvic floor yoga unfold with time. It's like watering that seed daily, providing it with the nourishment it needs to grow and flourish.

In fact, the International Urogynecology Journal published a study in 2018 showing significant improvements in pelvic floor muscle strength and urinary incontinence in women who performed these exercises regularly over six months. It's like watching that seed sprout, and then slowly grow into a robust, thriving plant.

Pelvic Floor Strength and Sexual Function

But that's not all. A study published in Sex Health Journal in 2018 highlighted the link between pelvic floor muscle exercises and improved sexual function in postmenopausal women.

Pelvic Floor and Core Strength

The magic of the pelvic floor doesn't stop there. These muscles can significantly improve the core strength necessary for balance and stability. For a visual, let's go back to the subway and it is much like adding more support pillars to your subway tunnels, making them stronger and more stable.

A study published in the Journal of Physical Therapy Science in 2015 found that pelvic floor muscle exercises improved balance and mobility in elderly women. This is so important for seniors! In my nursing career, I worked in long-term care. Fall prevention programs are at the forefront because the risk of falls increases with age and medical conditions. Falls are way too common for seniors. Unfortunately if falls result in significant or severe outcomes, this affects a person's daily functioning and quality of life.

I remember a resident who really struggled with the transition to long-term care after she fractured her shoulder due to falling. She had to move to long-term care for assistance. Before this, she had been fairly independent living in her home. She was struggling with the emotions of losing her independence and the need to rely on help from others for basic care such as toileting and bathing. She shared with me her feelings of losing control and autonomy and how receiving care affected her dignity and pride.

So, as you can see, your pelvic floor is a lot more than just a group of muscles. It's a vital part of your body's infrastructure, playing a crucial role in your overall health and wellbeing. It's about time we gave it the attention and care it deserves, don't you think?

Pelvic Floor Yoga: A Chair-Based Approach

Pelvic Floor Yoga: A Gentle Yet Powerful Practice

Chair-based pelvic floor yoga exercises are specifically designed to strengthen the pelvic floor, even for those with mobility limitations. It's like installing an elevator in your subway system, making it accessible to everyone, regardless of physical abilities.

These exercises involve contracting and relaxing the pelvic floor muscles, which can be done while seated. It's like performing a gentle dance with your muscles, right there in your chair.

So, are you ready to hop on this subway and explore the fascinating world of pelvic floor yoga? All you need is a chair, a bit of time, and the willingness to discover your body's inner strength. Your pelvic floor muscles might be hidden from view, but their impact on your health and well-being is definitely worth noticing. So, let's get started, one contraction, one relaxation, one breath at a time.

Your chair is waiting, your body is ready, and your journey into the heart of chair yoga is about to get even more exciting. So, hop on board, hold on tight, and let's enjoy this ride together!

Embrace the Power of Pelvic Floor Yoga from Your Chair

The Magic of Chair-Based Pelvic Floor Yoga

Isn't it amazing that a chair can transform into a personal gym? It's time to experience the magic of chair-based pelvic floor yoga. Designed with love and understanding for seniors and beginners, these exercises are all about improving the strength of your pelvic floor. Think of your chair as a cozy cocoon, providing support and stability as you gently work out those hidden pelvic muscles.

Contract and Relax: The Anthem of Pelvic Floor Yoga

What's the secret sauce of these exercises, you ask? Well, the mantra is simple: contract and relax. Imagine playing an accordion. You draw it in, then let it expand, playing a melodious tune. That's how you work your pelvic floor muscles - contract, then relax. And the sweet melody? That's the feeling of strength and control you develop over time.

Accessible Exercises for All

The best part about these exercises is their accessibility. Whether you're a sprightly senior or a yoga newbie, you can practice pelvic floor yoga right from the comfort of your chair. It's like having a universal key, opening doors for everyone, regardless of age or ability.

The Urology Care Foundation's Seal of Approval

But don't just take my word for it. The Urology Care Foundation, a leading authority in urologic health, recommends pelvic floor exercises for improving bladder control. It's like getting a thumbs up from a trusted friend, reinforcing your faith in the power of these exercises.

Pelvic Floor Yoga: A Part of Your Daily Routine

The beauty of pelvic floor yoga is that it can seamlessly blend into your daily routine. It's like adding a pinch of salt to a recipe, enhancing the flavor without overpowering it. You can practice these exercises while watching your favorite TV show, during ad breaks, or even while waiting for your morning coffee to brew.

Chair yoga is a unique, effective, and accessible approach to improving your pelvic floor strength. It's not just about the poses or the stretches; it's about focusing on those hidden muscles that play such a crucial role in your health and well-being.

It's time to give your pelvic floor muscles the attention they deserve. It's time to explore the power of chair-based pelvic floor yoga. So, get comfy in your chair, take a deep breath, and let's get started. Here's to stronger muscles, better control, and a healthier you!

Finding and Flexing: Locating Your Pelvic Floor

Unveiling the Mystery: Locating Your Pelvic Floor Muscles

Before we dive into the exercises, let's take a moment to locate our pelvic floor muscles. It's like going on a treasure hunt, with the treasure being your own body's hidden strength. The muscles that you use to hold in your urine and bowel movements are your pelvic floor muscles. Knowing that function can help you identify them.

Playing the Accordion: Contracting and Relaxing Your Pelvic Floor

Once you've located your pelvic floor muscles, you're ready to start exercising them. Remember the accordion analogy? Now's the time to play that sweet tune. Contract your muscles, then let them relax. It's like playing a gentle tug-of-war with yourself, pulling in, then letting go.

Breathing: The Rhythm of Pelvic Floor Yoga

And what about breathing, you ask? Well, your breath is the rhythm of your pelvic floor yoga dance. Make sure to breathe normally as you contract and relax your muscles. It's like the steady beat of a drum, guiding your movements and keeping you focused. Sometimes we tend to hold our breath when we're concentrating and focusing on something subtle. Keep breathing! It can be helpful to inhale and contract your pelvic floor muscles. Then exhale, and release the contraction.

No Pain, No Strain: The Golden Rule of Pelvic Floor Yoga

One crucial thing to remember is that pelvic floor yoga should never cause discomfort or pain. If it does, it's your body's way of saying you're pushing too hard or doing the exercises incorrectly. It's like your body's safety alarm, alerting you to stop and adjust your movements.

Consistency is Key: Making Pelvic Floor Yoga a Habit

The Power of Regular Practice

When it comes to pelvic floor yoga, consistency is key. It is finding a new language with your body. You wouldn't become fluent overnight with learning an entirely new language, would you? But with regular practice, you'd slowly but surely start understanding and speaking the language.

The National Association for Continence recommends performing pelvic floor exercises three times a day for the best results. So set regular dates with your pelvic floor muscles, spending quality time strengthening and toning them.

Monitor Your Progress: The Joy of Seeing Results

As you embark on this pelvic floor yoga journey, take a moment every now and then to look back and appreciate how far you've come. If you don't stop to give yourself credit for the small wins daily - who else will? This is an important life practice to pause, enjoy the view, and acknowledge your progress.

Keeping a journal can be a wonderful way to track your progress. Each entry serves as a mini-milestone, a snapshot of your journey. Note any improvements in bladder control, core strength, or balance. Use it to record the highlights of your journey and then you can look back on it and see how far you've come. These small but significant victories serve as a reminder of your growth and resilience.

Celebrate Small Wins: Keeping the Motivation Alive

And don't forget to celebrate your progress, no matter how small. Did you manage to hold your pelvic floor lift for a few seconds longer? That's a win. Did you notice an improvement in your bladder control? That's another win. Each small win is a step towards your overall goal, an affirmation of your hard work and dedication. Learn to appreciate every moment of growth and progress.

Each small win in your pelvic floor yoga practice is a cherished souvenir, a testament to your efforts and achievements.

So, get ready to embrace the power of pelvic floor yoga. Your chair is waiting, your body is ready, and a whole new world of strength and control is just a contraction away. Here's to a stronger, healthier, and happier you!

Now, let's continue our chair yoga adventure, exploring more poses, more benefits, and more surprises. Stay tuned, keep practicing, and let's enjoy this exciting journey together.

How to Do Pelvic Floor Yoga from Your Chair

Identifying Your Pelvic Floor Muscles

First things first, let's get familiar with the star of the show - your pelvic floor muscles. These muscles are subtle but powerful, like an ancient hidden treasure. The first step? Locating the treasure. Similarly, before we start exercising our pelvic floor muscles, we need to find them.

Here's a simple trick recommended by the Mayo Clinic: try pausing your pee mid-flow. The muscles you engage to do this are your pelvic floor muscles. Now, remember, this is just to help you identify the muscles. Regularly stopping your pee can interfere with bladder function, and we definitely don't want that. This is called the Stop-test. **Only** do this if you have no awareness of your pelvic floor muscles.

Contract and Release: The Pelvic Floor Dance

Now that we've found our treasure, it's time to shine it up. The key to pelvic floor exercises is a simple 'contract and release' pattern. Think of it as a dance with your pelvic floor muscles.

To get started, sit comfortably in your chair, feet flat on the ground. Now, imagine you're pulling up your pelvic floor muscles into your body, like an elevator going up. Hold this contraction for a few seconds, then slowly lower the elevator back down, releasing the contraction. That's it - you've just done your first pelvic floor exercise!

Quick Flicks for a Quick Workout

Got the hang of the pelvic floor lift? Great! Now let's add another move to our pelvic floor dance - quick flicks. Picture yourself playing a snappy tune on a piano. The keys are your pelvic floor muscles, and the tune is a quick succession of notes.

While seated, quickly lift and lower your pelvic floor muscles, as if you're playing those fast notes on a piano. Do this a few times, always making sure to keep breathing normally. Remember, these exercises should never cause discomfort or pain. So, if it doesn't feel right, take a break and try again later.

Breathe Easy: The Pelvic Floor Mantra

Speaking of breathing, let's not forget the importance of breath in pelvic floor yoga. Nature is a good example. Just like the gentle rise and fall of a butterfly's wings, that's how your breath should flow - gentle, rhythmical, and effortless.

During your pelvic floor exercises, make sure to keep your breath steady and relaxed. There's no need to hold your breath or to breathe in any particular pattern. Just let your breath flow naturally, like that butterfly in the garden.

Gentle and Easy Does It

One golden rule of pelvic floor yoga is to always prioritize comfort over intensity. It's not about how hard you can push yourself, but about how gently and consistently you can exercise your muscles. If you feel any discomfort or strain, it's a sign that you're pushing too hard. So, ease off a bit and remember, gentle and easy does it!

This is a simple, yet effective beginning to practicing pelvic floor yoga from your chair. It's not about grand movements or complicated poses. It's about subtle, gentle exercises that can strengthen your pelvic floor muscles, improve your core strength, and enhance your overall health.

So, pull up your favorite chair, take a deep breath, and let's get moving. Here's to a stronger, healthier pelvic floor, one contraction, one release, one breath at a time.

Making Pelvic Floor Yoga a Habit: A Routine to Rejoice

Consistency: The Secret Ingredient

Let's face it, magic potions and quick-fix solutions only exist in fairy tales. In the real world, especially when it comes to fitness, it's consistency that weaves the true magic. It's like watering a plant regularly. You don't see the results instantly, but over time, that tiny seedling grows into a robust, blooming plant.

As mentioned, The National Association for Continence, a leading resource in bladder health, advises doing pelvic floor exercises three times a day for the most beneficial results. It's like having three fitness dates with your pelvic floor muscles every day - a morning coffee date, an afternoon catch-up, and an evening wind-down.

Integrating Pelvic Floor Yoga into Your Daily Routine: Seamless and Simple

Now, you might be thinking, "Three times a day? That's a lot!" But here's the wonderful thing about pelvic floor yoga - it can be effortlessly woven into your daily routine. It's like adding a dash of spice to your favorite dish. It doesn't overpower the dish; it simply enhances the flavor.

You can do these exercises while binge-watching your favorite TV show, waiting for your oven to preheat, or even grooming in the bathroom. It's a way to turn your idle moments into opportunities for fitness and well-being.

Age is Just a Number: It's Never Too Late to Start

And remember, it's never too late to start exercising your pelvic floor muscles. Whether you're a sprightly senior, a yoga newbie, or somewhere in between, chair-based pelvic floor yoga is accessible and beneficial for everyone. It's like learning to swim. It doesn't matter how old you are or how deep the water is. What matters is your willingness to try, to learn, and to keep going, one stroke at a time.

So now you have a simple yet effective routine to strengthen your pelvic floor muscles, right from the comfort of your chair. It's not just about the exercises; it's about the consistency, the progress, the celebration of small wins, and the joy of discovering your body's hidden strength.

So, why wait? Your chair is ready, your body is excited, and a whole new world of strength and control is waiting to be discovered.

As our exploration of chair yoga continues, we'll delve deeper into the fascinating world of poses, benefits, and surprises that this practice holds. So, stay tuned, keep practicing, and let's continue this exciting adventure together.

Let's now gear up for the next chapter where we will delve into the world of yoga poses that are not just fun and relaxing but also incredibly effective for weight loss. So, stay tuned, keep practicing, and let's continue this exciting journey together.

CHAPTER EIGHT

RISE AND SHINE

MORNING CHAIR YOGA FOR A BRIGHTER DAY

It's a brand-new day, full of promise and potential. And, instead of hitting the snooze button and burrowing back under the covers, what if you could start your day with an invigorating chair yoga routine? A routine that wakes you up better than any cup of coffee, fills you up with positive energy and sets you up for a day of success and well-being. Intrigued? Buckle up, my friend, because we're about to turn your mornings from groggy to glorious!

The Wake-Up-With-Yoga Routine: A Good Morning Indeed

Pull up your favorite chair, take a deep breath, and let's dive into a morning routine that will raise your energy and give you a boost to start your day. Some of these poses have already been covered in previous chapters. This chapter will give you a perfect morning routine of the chair yoga poses to give you a great foundation to start your day.

Energizing Breathwork

Wake Up, Lungs!

Begin your morning chair yoga with a simple yet powerful breathing exercise. It's like giving your lungs a wake-up call, preparing them for the day ahead.

Sit comfortably in your chair, spine straight, and eyes closed. Take a slow, deep breath in through your nose, filling your lungs with fresh morning air. Hold your breath for a few seconds, then exhale slowly, releasing all the air out. Repeat this deep breathing for a few rounds, feeling your body wake up with each breath.

Morning Stretch Sequence

Gentle Neck Rolls

Next, let's wake up those neck muscles with some gentle neck rolls. It's like doing a slow dance with your neck, loosening up those stiff muscles.

Sit tall in your chair, relax your shoulders, and lower your right ear towards your right shoulder. Slowly roll your head towards the front, bringing your chin to your chest. Continue rolling your head towards the left, bringing your left ear towards your left shoulder. Repeat this gentle neck roll a few times, then switch directions.

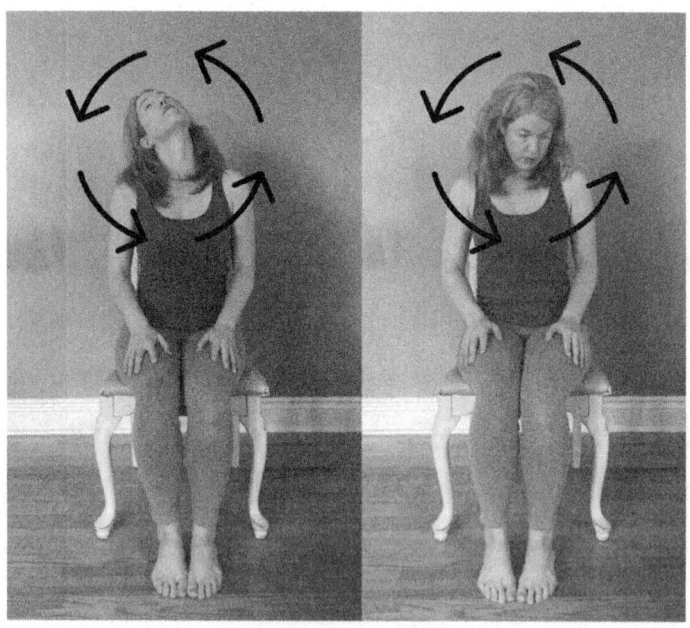

Gentle Neck Rolls

Seated Side Stretches

Now, let's stretch out those sides with a seated side stretch. Imagine you're a willow tree, swaying gracefully in the morning breeze.

Sit tall in your chair, feet flat on the ground. As you inhale, reach your right arm up towards the ceiling. As you exhale, lean your torso towards the left, feeling a nice stretch along the right side of your body. Inhale back to the center, then repeat on the other side.

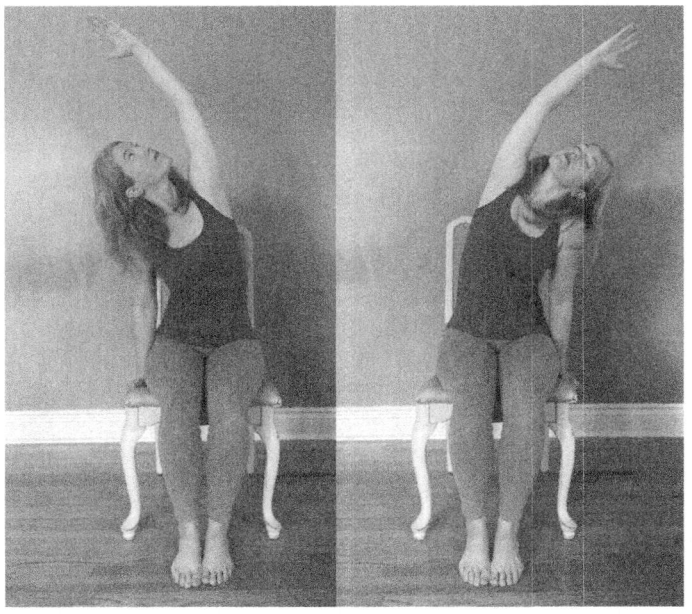

Seated Side Stretches

Seated Twist

Next up, let's add a twist to our morning stretch sequence. Picture yourself wringing out a wet towel, releasing all the tension and stiffness from your body.

Sit tall in your chair, feet flat on the ground. Place your right hand on your left knee and your left hand on the backrest of your chair. As you inhale, lengthen your spine, and as you exhale, gently twist your upper body towards the left. Inhale back to the center, then repeat on the other side.

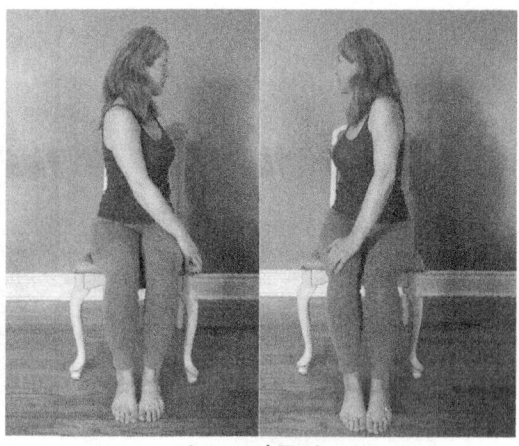

Seated Twist

Poses for Mental Clarity

Chair Eagle Pose

Now, it's time to clear the morning fog from our minds with the Chair Eagle Pose. Imagine yourself as an eagle, soaring high above the clouds, enjoying a clear, panoramic view of the world below.

While seated, extend your arms in front of you. Cross your right arm over the left, then bend your elbows and wrap your forearms around each other, bringing your palms together. Hold this pose for a few breaths, feeling a nice stretch in your shoulders and upper back. Unwind your arms, then repeat with the left arm crossed over the right.

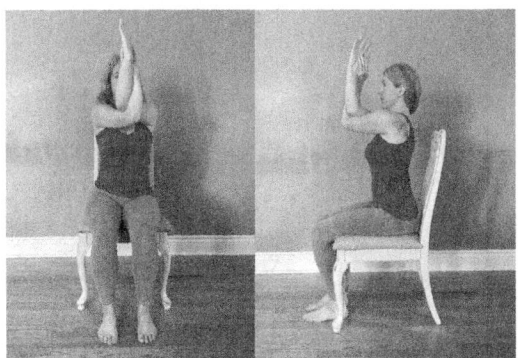

Eagle Arms

Chair Mountain Pose

Finally, let's ground ourselves for the day ahead with the Chair Mountain Pose. Picture yourself as a towering mountain, stable, strong, and serene.

Sit tall in your chair, feet flat on the ground, hands resting on your thighs. Imagine a string attached to the top of your head, pulling you up towards the ceiling. Feel the stability in your body, the calmness in your mind. Hold this pose for a few breaths, basking in the tranquility of the moment.

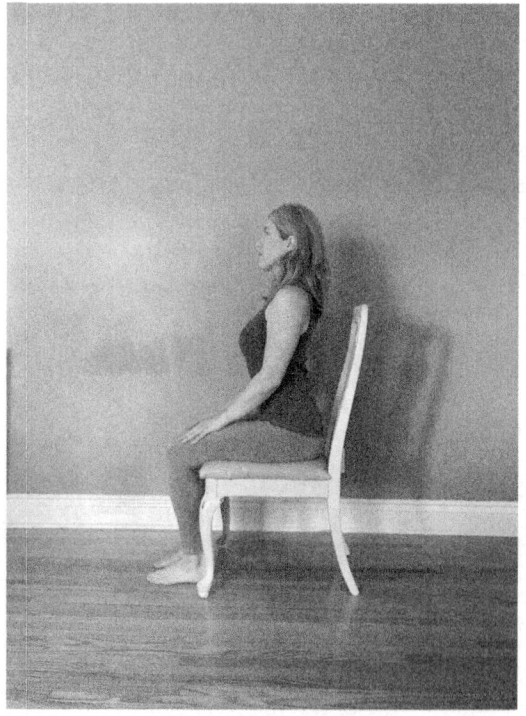

Mountain Pose

So now you have a refreshing morning chair yoga routine that's sure to put a spring in your step and a sparkle in your eye. It's the perfect way to greet the day, energize your body, and clear your mind – all from the comfort of your chair. So, go ahead, and give it a try tomorrow morning. Your body will thank you for it, and who knows, you might just become a morning person after all!

How to Do Yoga in Your Pajamas: Comfort Meets Fitness

Gentle Seated Poses: The Perfect Morning Stretch

Imagine waking up, rubbing the sleep out of your eyes, and instead of reaching for that cup of coffee, you reach for your... chair? Yes, indeed! Welcome to a morning like no other, where comfort meets fitness in a glorious blend of chair yoga. No need to change out of your pajamas; they're the perfect attire for a comfy yoga session.

Let's start with the Seated Tadasana or the Mountain Pose. This pose is all about grounding yourself and setting the tone for the day. Sit on your chair with your feet flat on the ground and your spine straight. Rest your hands on your thighs, close your eyes, and take a few deep breaths. Feel the calm seeping into your body with each breath, washing away any remnants of sleep. See the image above.

Next, transition into the Chair Cat-Cow Stretch. This pose is about waking up your spine and saying goodbye to any stiffness. Place your hands on your knees. As you inhale, arch your back and lift your chest towards the ceiling. As you exhale, round your back and drop your chin towards your chest. Repeat this a few times, moving with your breath.

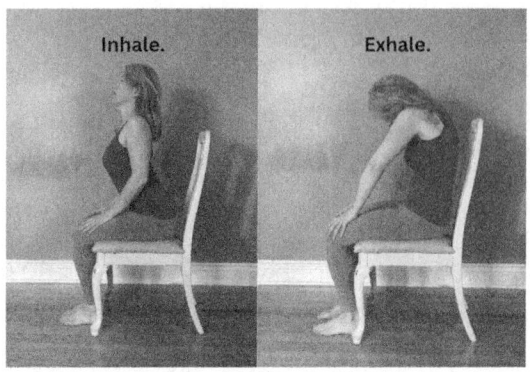

Seated Cat and Cow

Relaxing Breathwork: A Gentle Wake-Up Call

Now that your body is awake, let's wake up your lungs with some relaxing breathwork. Think of it as a gentle morning whisper, rousing your body from its slumber.

Start with the Full Yogic Breath, a simple yet powerful technique that maximizes your oxygen intake. Inhale deeply into your belly, then your rib cage, and finally your chest. As you exhale, release the breath from your chest, then your rib cage, and finally your belly. Repeat this a few times, feeling your body fill up with fresh morning air.

Next, try the Bee Breath or Bhramari Pranayama. This technique is like a soothing lullaby for your nervous system. Close your eyes, take a deep breath in, and as you exhale, make a humming sound, like a bee. Feel the vibration of the sound calming your mind and body.

Mindful Meditation Techniques: Starting Your Day on a Positive Note

With your body and breath awake, let's wake up your mind with some mindful meditation. It's like greeting the morning sun, filling your mind with its warm, golden light.

Start with a simple mindfulness practice. Sit comfortably in your chair, close your eyes, and bring your attention to your breath. Notice the sensation of the breath entering and leaving your body. If your mind wanders, gently bring it back to your breath. It's like watching the waves on a beach, coming in and going out.

Next, try a gratitude meditation. Think of three things you're grateful for. It could be as simple as the comfort of your bed, the taste of your morning coffee, or the roof over your head. Feel the gratitude filling your heart, and let it set a positive tone for your day.

You now have a morning chair yoga routine that you can do in your pajamas. It's gentle, relaxing, and the perfect way to start your day. So, go ahead, roll out of bed, pull up a chair, and give it a try. After all, who said you can't have a fitness routine in your pajamas?

Now, let's continue our exploration of chair yoga. We've got more poses, more techniques, and more surprises in store for you.

The Early Bird's Guide to Chair Yoga

Waking up early has its own set of advantages, and for all you early birds out there, we've got an exciting and energizing chair yoga routine lined up for you. This routine is all about greeting the sunrise with vitality, balance, and a dash of exuberance. So, let's roll up our sleeves and get started!

Sunrise Salutation Sequence

What better way to start your morning than by saluting the rising sun? The Sunrise Salutation Sequence was covered in Chapter 6 and it is a modified version of the traditional Sun Salutation, adapted for chair yoga. It's a series of poses performed in a flowing sequence, designed to energize your body and awaken your senses. It is perfect to do upon rising as part of your morning yoga practice.

Begin by sitting upright on your chair, feet flat on the ground. As you inhale, sweep your arms out to the sides and overhead, reaching for the sky. As you exhale, bring your hands to the heart center, then fold forward over your legs leading with your chest, letting your hands rest on your shins or the floor.

Inhale, lift your torso halfway, extending your spine and looking forward. Exhale, and fold forward once again. Inhale, sweep your arms out to the sides and overhead, coming back to the starting position. Exhale, bring your hands back to the heart center. Repeat this sequence a few times, moving with your breath.

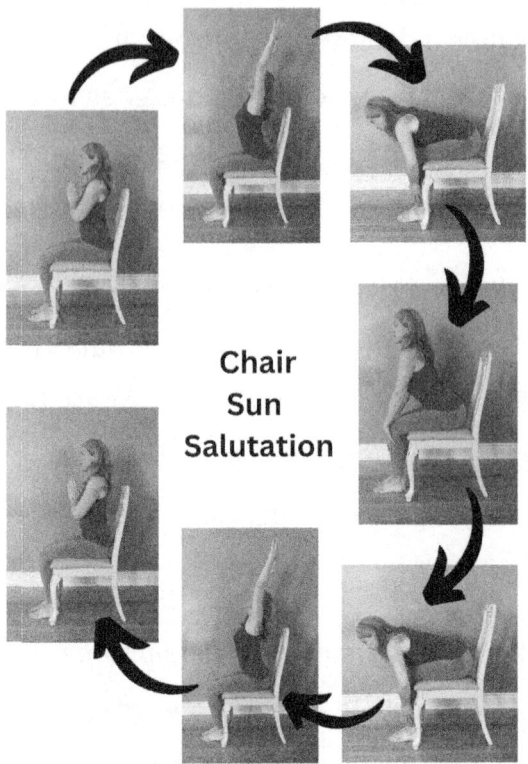

Chair Sun Salutation

Poses for Balance and Stability

Once you've warmed up your body with the Sunrise Salutation, let's move on to some poses that focus on balance and stability. These poses are like the roots of a tree, providing a strong and stable foundation for your day.

First up, we have the Chair Warrior II Pose. Sit sideways on your chair, your right leg bent at the knee, and your left leg extended straight out behind you. Extend your arms out to the sides, turning your head to look over your front hand. Feel your body aligning with your breath, like a warrior standing strong and steady.

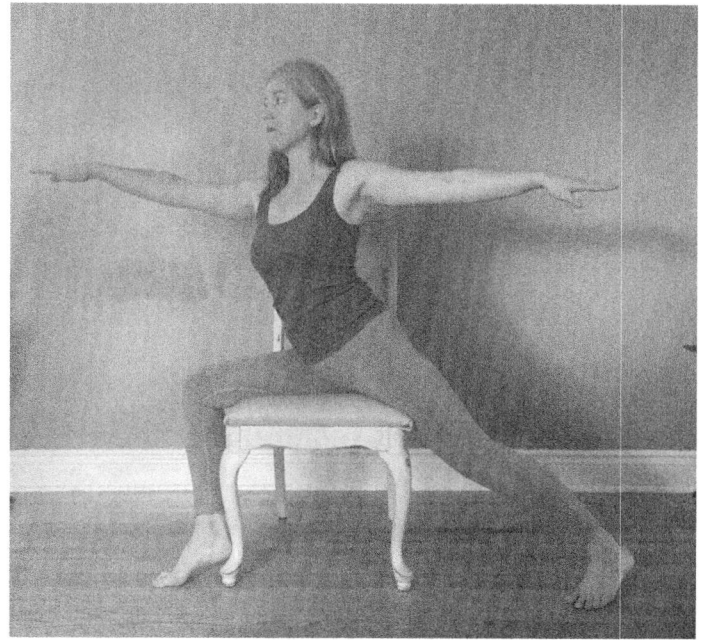

Chair Warrior II Pose

Next, let's try the Chair Tree Pose. While seated, place your right foot on the inside of your left leg, either above or below the knee. Bring your hands to the heart center, focusing on a point in front of you for balance. Feel the stability in your body, like a tree standing tall and firm.

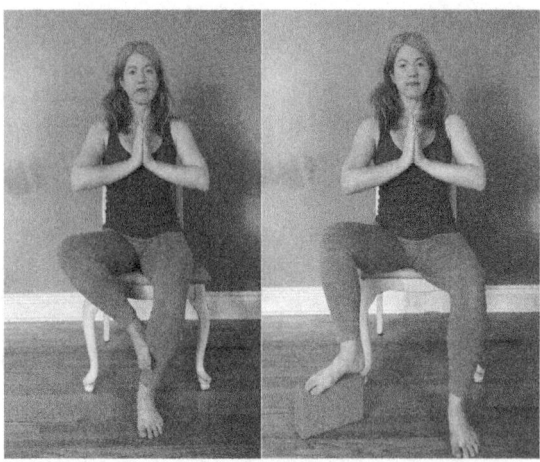

*Chair Tree Pose and Variation Supported
with Block*

Energizing Breathwork Techniques

To round off your morning routine, let's engage in some energizing breathwork techniques. These techniques are like a fresh cup of coffee, awakening your senses and preparing you for the day ahead.

Bellows Breath

Start with the Bellows Breath, or Bhastrika Pranayama. This technique involves rapid, forceful breaths in and out through your nose. It's like fanning a flame, stoking your body's energy and vitality.

Breath of Fire

Next, let's try the Breath of Fire, or Kapalabhati Pranayama. This technique involves short, sharp exhales through your nose, with passive inhales. The emphasis is on the exhale through your nostrils while pulling the navel point in. The inhale happens naturally as the belly relaxes out. This powerful breathwork generates heat in the body and is detoxifying. Do not practice this breath if you have had recent abdominal surgery or trauma. Also do not do this breath if you are pregnant or menstruating.

Laughing Breath

Lastly, let's try the Laughing Breath, a technique that's as fun as it sounds. Simply take a deep breath in, then exhale with a hearty laugh. It may feel forced at first but when you really let yourself go and fake the laugh, sometimes it catches on and erupts into a cathartic release. Laughing works the core and pelvic floor muscles!

These breathwork techniques are not just about breathing in and out. They're about awakening your body's energy, preparing you for a day of success and well-being. So, the next time you wake up early, try this chair yoga routine. It's sure to put a spring in your step and a twinkle in your eye. Here's to an energizing start to your day!

Starting Your Day with a Yoga Smile: Positivity at Its Best

Poses for Positive Energy

Let's kickstart with a few poses that fill you up with positivity and energy.

Seated Sun Pose

First off, we have the Seated Sun Pose, a stretch that radiates positivity from head to toe. Picture a sunflower reaching out to the morning sun, soaking up the golden light. That's the vibe we're aiming for!

Sit comfortably in your chair, feet flat on the ground. As you inhale, raise your arms overhead, stretching your body towards the ceiling. As you exhale, gently lean to the right, feeling a nice stretch on your left side. Inhale back to the center, then repeat on the other side.

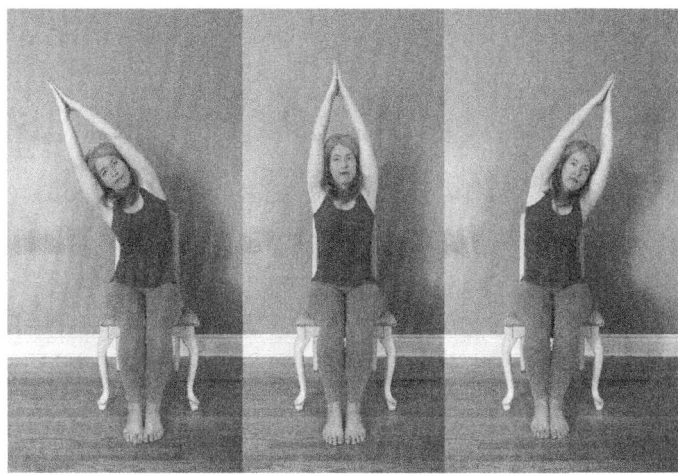

Seated Sun Pose

Chair Happy Pose

Next, we have the Chair Happy Pose, a pose that's all about embracing joy and shedding off any morning blues. Imagine a baby giggling with pure, unfiltered joy. That's the energy we're channeling in this pose.

While seated, hug your right knee into your chest, wrapping your arms around your shin. Hold for a few breaths, feeling a gentle stretch in your hip. Release and repeat with the other leg.

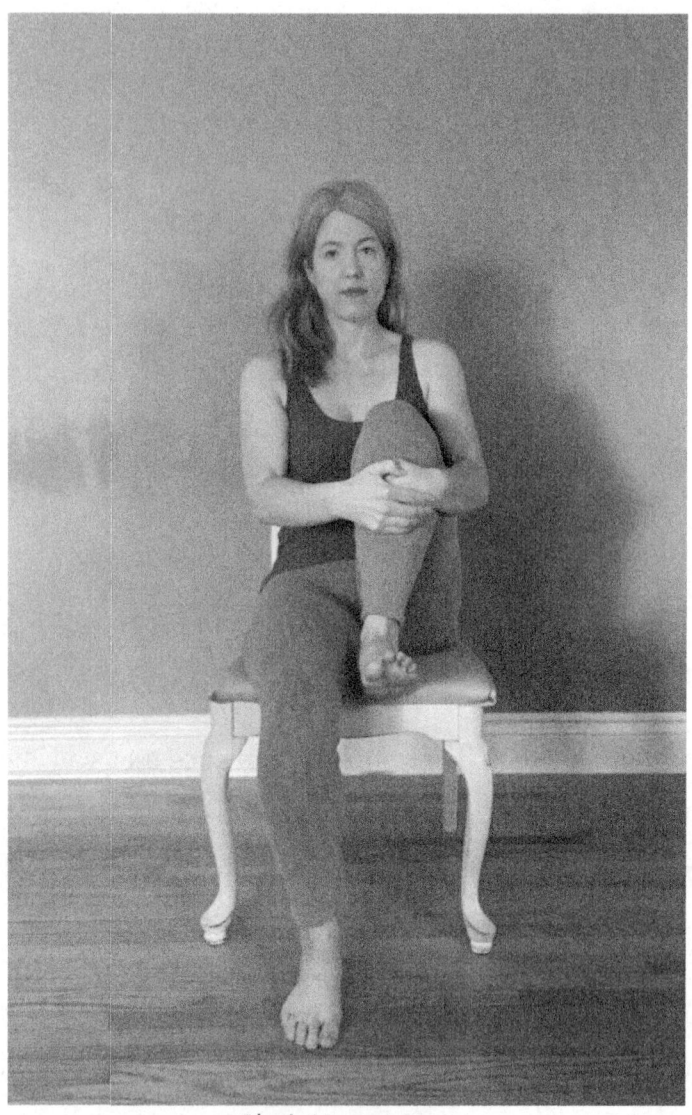

Chair Happy Pose

Chair Hip Circles

To build on the last pose, Chair Happy pose, we will move into hip circles. Sit tall on your chair. Hold that right leg up from the hip. Challenge yourself and see if you can hold that right leg up without placing your hands on it. Trace circles in the air with that right knee moving clockwise from your hips. Then change direction. When you're done with the right leg, repeat the hip circles in both directions on the left side. If you're not holding on to your leg, it can be helpful to place your hands on the edges of the seat to help stabilize you.

So, you now have a morning chair yoga routine that promises to add a dash of positivity, a sprinkle of joy, and a whole lot of smiles to your day. From energizing poses and calming meditations to uplifting breathwork, each element of this routine is designed to help you start your day on a high note.

As we continue to explore the wonders of chair yoga, we'll discover more poses, delve deeper into breathwork, and learn how to make the most of this incredible practice. So, stay tuned, keep smiling, and let's make every day a chair yoga day!

CHAPTER NINE

EMBRACE THE NIGHT

UNWINDING WITH CHAIR YOGA FOR BETTER SLEEP

"Twinkle, twinkle, little star, how I wonder what you are." Remember this nursery rhyme from our childhood? As we grow older, we might not gaze at stars with the same wonder (although seeing a clear night sky still takes my breath away). For most grown-ups, there's a different kind of twinkle we yearn for - the twinkle of peaceful sleep. If you're someone who spends more time awake at 3 a.m. with your worries than actually sleeping, then you're in the right place. We're about to discover how chair yoga can help you snooze like a baby and wake up feeling as fresh as a daisy.

The moon has risen, the day's hustle and bustle is behind you and now it's time to unwind. Your faithful chair is waiting, ready to support you in a series of relaxing yoga poses designed to prepare your body and mind for a good night's sleep. Remember you may have seen some of these poses throughout the book. This chapter specifically focuses on poses that are best to do before bed.

Evening Yoga Poses for Sweeter Dreams

Chair Child's Pose: The Cocoon of Comfort

You get to curl up like a caterpillar and snuggle in a cozy cocoon, safe and comfortable. That's what we're emulating with the Chair Child's Pose.

Here's how you do it:

- Start by sitting midway on your chair, feet flat on the floor.

- Spread your knees wide while keeping your big toes touching.

- Now, fold forward from your hips, letting your torso rest between your thighs.

- Stretch your arms out in front of you, resting your forearms on the chair or letting them hang towards the floor.

- For extra support you can place a couple of pillows on your lap or a pillow and a block to support your upper body.

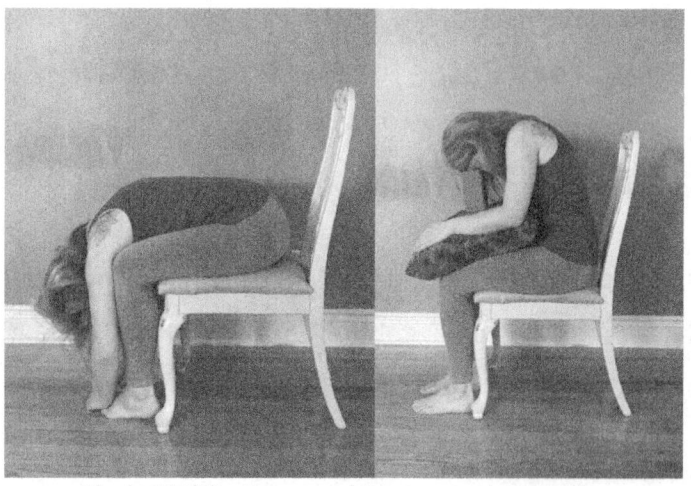

Chair Child's Pose and Supported Variation

This pose is like a warm hug to your body, a signal that it's time to relax and let go. As you breathe in this pose, imagine each exhale releasing the day's stress, worries, and fatigue. You will feel a release in your lower back and an opening up in your hips.

Seated Forward Bend: The Gentle Goodnight

Remember how, as kids, we'd bend down to say goodnight to our pet dog or cat before hopping into bed? The Seated Forward Bend is a similar goodnight signal to your body, only this time, we're saying goodnight to the day.

Here's how you do it:

- Sit tall on your chair, feet flat on the floor.

- Inhale deeply, lifting your arms up overhead.

- As you exhale, hinge from your hips and bend forward, leading with your chest.

- Let your hands rest on your legs, feet, or the floor, whichever feels comfortable.

As you stay in this pose, let go of any tension in your neck and shoulders. It's like you're gently shaking off the day, preparing your body for a peaceful night's sleep.

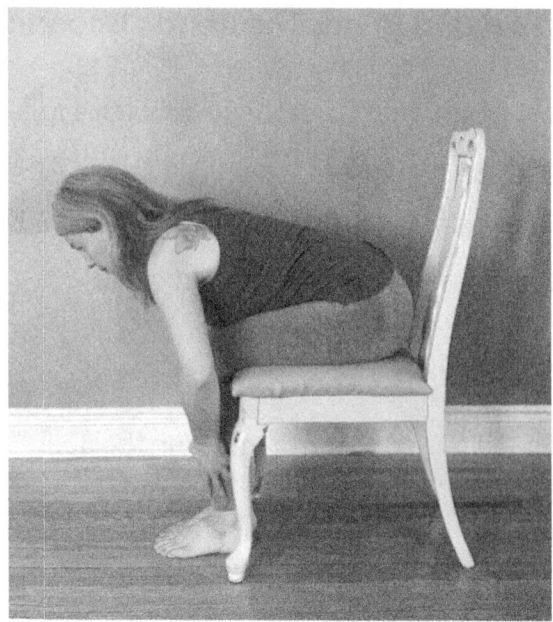

Seated Forward Bend

Chair Savasana: The Star of the Night

Finally, we come to Chair Savasana, the star of our nighttime yoga routine. If our yoga session was a night sky, Savasana would be the brightest star, signaling the end of the day and the beginning of a serene night.

Here's how you do it:

- Sit back comfortably in your chair, allowing it to support your body.

- Rest your hands on your thighs or let them hang by your sides.

- Close your eyes and breathe naturally.

As you stay in this pose, imagine your body becoming light, like a feather floating in the night sky. Every muscle, every cell in your body is switching into sleep mode, ready to rejuvenate through the night.

This is a good start to having a sequence of relaxing chair yoga poses to help you wind down and set the stage for a peaceful slumber. Remember, the key lies in the breath. As you move through these poses, let your breath be your guide, slow and steady, like the quiet rhythm of the night. Here's to sweeter dreams, and restful nights with chair yoga. Sweet dreams!

The Night Owl's Guide to Chair Yoga

Congratulations, fellow night owl! You've chosen to end your day on a tranquil note, and chair yoga is ready to accompany you on this serene voyage. When the moon is high, and most are tucked away in the realm of dreams, we can create a quiet sanctuary of relaxation right on our chairs. Let's explore how we can lull our bodies into a state of tranquility, one pose, and one breath at a time.

Gentle Stretching Sequence: The Nighttime Ballet

Let's begin with a sequence of gentle stretches that will help release the tension from your body. These exercises and stretches will allow you to bid farewell to the day's stress.

Start with a Seated Side Stretch. As you sit tall on your chair, raise your right arm overhead, reaching for the stars. With your next exhale, gently lean to your left, imagining yourself as a willow tree swaying gently in the night breeze.

Then do the other side and raise your left arm overhead with the inhale. On the exhale, gently lean to the right. You can feel that stretch on the side of your body. Enjoy!

Next, transition into a Chair Seated Spinal Twist. As you sit tall, place your right hand on your left knee and gently twist your upper body to the left. With each exhale, deepen the twist, wringing out the day's worries from your mind. Then twist to the left to balance out the other side.

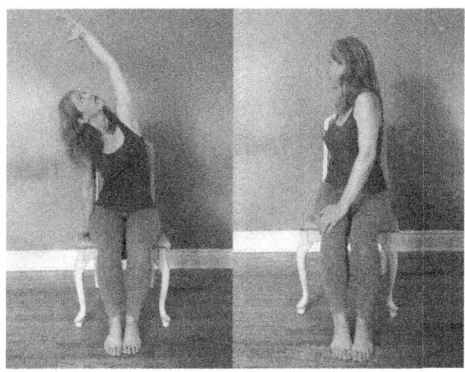

Finally, let's do a Chair Leg Lift to stretch out those tired legs. While seated, extend your right leg out in front of you, flexing your foot. Feel the stretch in your hamstring, like a silent yawn after a long day. With your foot extended, start circling your ankles in a clockwise direction. Then circle your ankle in the other direction. Remember to switch legs and give your left leg the same sweet stretch and also give it some loving ankle circles.

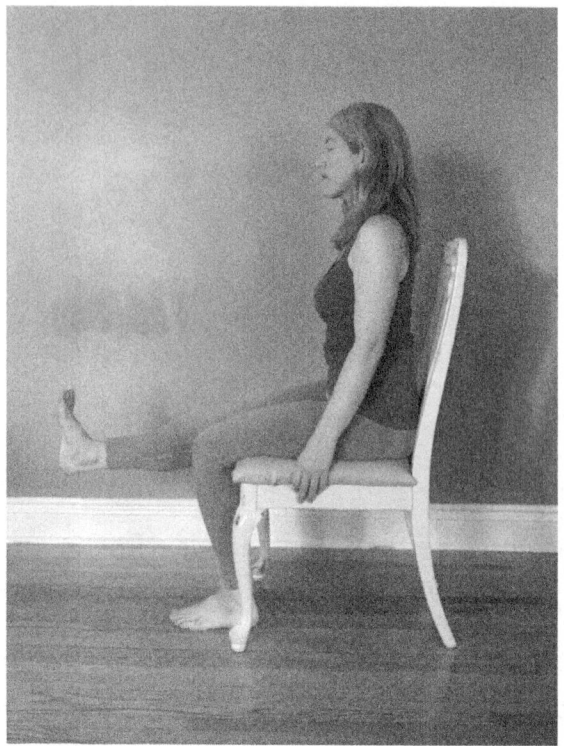

Chair Leg Lift

Relaxing Breathwork Techniques: The Nighttime Symphony

Now that your body is stretched and relaxed, let's tune into the rhythm of our breath. It's your body's own nighttime symphony, with each breath playing a soothing note.

Begin with the 4-7-8 Breathing Technique. Inhale for a count of 4, hold your breath for a count of 7, then exhale for a count of 8. This rhythmic breathing can help slow down your heart rate, preparing your body for sleep.

Next, let's revisit the Box Breathing Technique. Inhale, hold, exhale, and hold again, each for a count of 4. It's like drawing a square in the air with your breath, bringing a sense of balance and calm to your mind.

Mindful Meditation Practices: The Moonlit Path to Peace

Finally, let's end our nighttime chair yoga routine with some mindful meditation.

Start with a simple Body Scan Meditation. Close your eyes and bring your attention to the top of your head. Slowly move your awareness down your body, noticing any sensations, tension, or relaxation in each part. You can stop at each body part and acknowledge it. Saying, "Goodnight foot, it's okay to relax now." You can go through each part of your body, one at a time.

Next, let's practice some Loving-Kindness Meditation. Think of someone you care about, and silently send them love and good wishes. You can focus on your heart center and fill it with light. This light can be any color, whatever color first comes. As you inhale, this light keeps expanding and filling your heart with warmth and love.

So, fellow night owl, here's your guide to a serene end to the day with chair yoga. May your nights be as peaceful as a tranquil lake under a starry sky, and may each morning greet you with renewed energy and joy. Sleep well and sweet dreams!

The Bedtime Chair Yoga Routine: A Lullaby for Your Body and Mind

Poses for Relaxation: Unwind and Let Go

As the moon takes up the night watch, it's time for your body to slide into a state of relaxation. That's the essence of these next few poses.

Seated Side Extended Angle Pose

Begin with the Seated Side Extended Angle Pose. This pose is all about side stretches that help release tension from your hips, lower back, middle back, hamstrings, and inner thighs. This pose also helps to open the channels for the easy flow of *prana* – life force energy.

Seated on the Chair: Inhale and place the left thigh on the chair seated sideways. Exhale and stretch the right leg out stretching the knee and ankle. Inhale and raise the right arm up above your head. Exhale and place the left arm to rest on the left thigh. Look up. Stay here for 3 complete yogic breaths. Release and relax. Then repeat with the right leg on the chair and stay for 3 breaths. Release and relax.

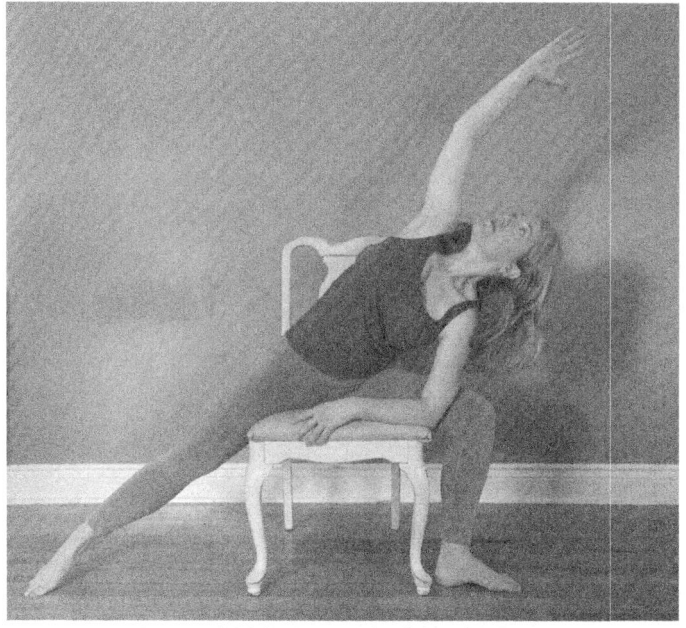

Seated Side Extended Angle Pose

Chair Reclining Bound Angle Pose

Next, transition into the Chair Reclining Bound Angle Pose. This pose is about opening up your hips and creating space in your chest.

While seated, bring the soles of your feet together, allowing your knees to fall out to the sides. Lean back in your chair, letting your backrest comfortably against the backrest. Place one hand on your heart and the other on your belly, feeling the rise and fall of your breath.

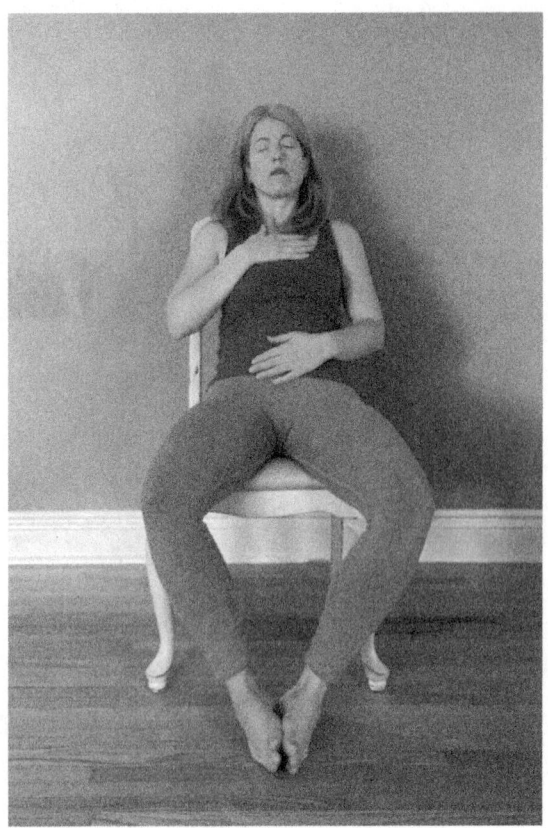

Chair Reclining Bound Angle

Gentle Stretching Sequence: A Serenade to Your Muscles

After the calming poses, let's serenade our muscles with a sequence of gentle stretches.

Chair Extended Hand-To-Big-Toe Pose

Start with the Chair Extended Hand-To-Big-Toe Pose. This pose is a gentle hamstring stretch that also challenges your balance.

While seated, extend your right leg out in front of you, holding your right big toe with your right hand. If you can't reach your toes, reach for your ankle or your shin. Do you best! Keep your left hand on your left hip for balance. Hold for a few breaths, then switch sides.

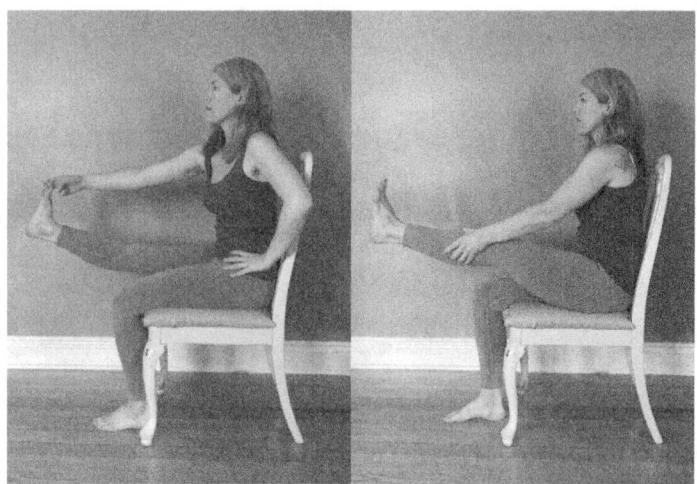

Hand-to-Big-Toe Pose

Breathwork for Sleep: The Gentle Whisper of the Night

As we wind down our bedtime chair yoga routine, let's tune into the gentle whisper of our breath. Use your breath to quiet your mind and soothe yourself to sleep.

Alternate Nostril Breathing

Begin with Alternate Nostril Breathing, a technique that balances your mind and prepares your body for sleep.

While seated, sit up straight with your feet flat on the floor. Lift your right hand and gently close your right nostril with your thumb. Inhale through your left nostril, then close it with your ring finger. Release your thumb and exhale through your right nostril. Then inhale through your right nostril, close it with your thumb, release your ring finger, and exhale through your left nostril. Repeat this sequence a few times, letting your breath flow like a gentle night breeze.

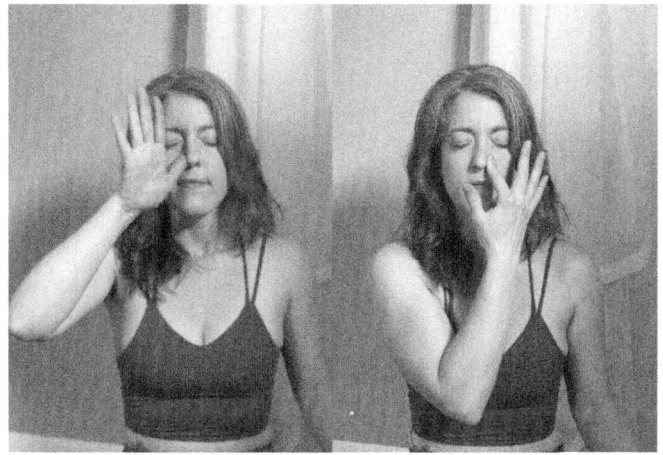

Alternate Nostril Breathing

Brahmari Breathing

Next, let's try Brahmari Breathing, also known as Bee Breathing. This technique is like the distant hum of a bee, calming your senses and promoting sleep.

Close your eyes and take a slow, deep breath in. As you exhale, make a humming sound, like a bee. Feel the vibration of the sound calming your mind, lulling you into a state of relaxation.

So, my dear friend, here's your ticket to a peaceful night's sleep - a sequence of relaxing poses, gentle stretches, and soothing breathwork, all from the comfort of your chair. As you practice these techniques, let the peace of the night envelop you, guiding you into a world of dreams. Goodnight, and sleep tight!

Sleep, Sweet Sleep: Using Chair Yoga to Combat Insomnia

Relaxing Seated Poses: The Magic Carpet Ride

Picture yourself on a magic carpet, floating effortlessly through a clear night sky, stars twinkling above, peace enveloping you. That's the state of relaxation we're aiming for with these seated poses. You are likely familiar with these poses already. They are the perfect complement to do right before sleep. So, hop onto your chair, your magic carpet for the night, and let's float away into a world of tranquility.

Let's begin with the Seated Side Bend, a pose that's all about releasing tension and embracing relaxation. Sit tall on your chair, feet flat on the ground. As you inhale, raise your right arm up towards the ceiling, and as you exhale, gently lean to your left, enjoying a delicious stretch along your right side.

Next, let's transition into the Seated Gentle Twist. While seated, place your right hand on your left knee and your left hand on the backrest of your chair. Take a deep breath in, and as you exhale, gently twist your upper body to the left, looking over your left shoulder.

Then make sure you do the side bend and the gentle twist on the other side. Yoga is all about balance.

These poses will wash away the day's stress, and carry you closer to a peaceful slumber.

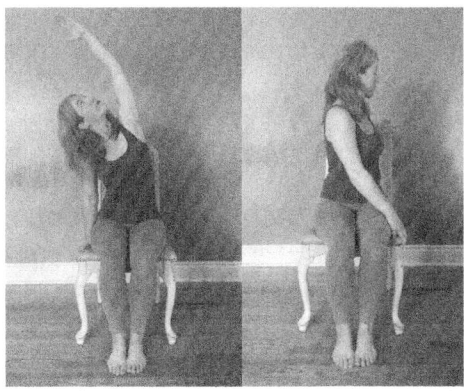

Breathwork for Calm: The Lullaby of Your Breath

Now that your body is relaxed, let's tune into the gentle rhythmic wave of your breath.

Begin with the Full Yogic Breath, a simple yet powerful technique that fills your body with calm. Close your eyes, take a slow, deep breath in, filling your belly, then your rib cage, and finally your chest. As you exhale, release the breath from your chest, then your rib cage, and finally your belly.

Next, let's try the Cooling Breath. This technique is like a soothing moonbeam, cooling your body and preparing it for sleep. Stick out your tongue and curl it into a tube. Inhale through your tongue, then close your mouth and exhale through your nose.

These breathwork techniques are not just about inhaling and exhaling. They're about weaving a blanket of tranquility around you, one breath at a time.

Mindful Meditation Techniques: A Moonlit Walk to Peace

Lastly, let's embark on a moonlit walk to peace with some mindful meditation techniques. It's like taking a leisurely stroll under the starry night sky, each step bringing you closer to a serene sleep.

Start with a simple Mindfulness Meditation. Sit comfortably in your chair, close your eyes, and bring your attention to your breath. Notice the cool air entering your nostrils and the warm air leaving. If your mind wanders, gently bring it back to your breath.

Next, let's try a Guided Imagery Meditation. Close your eyes and imagine a peaceful scene, like a quiet beach under the moonlight or a serene forest bathed in starlight. Immerse yourself in this scene, engaging all your senses.

These meditation techniques are like a quiet lullaby, gently guiding you towards a peaceful sleep.

So, my dear friend, let's bid farewell to sleepless nights and embrace the soothing world of chair yoga. Here's to a night of restful sleep, sweet dreams, and a morning full of renewed energy and joy. Goodnight and sleep tight!

As we continue to explore the wonders of chair yoga, tomorrow is a new day to discover more poses, techniques, and the surprising benefits that this practice holds. So, rest well, and we'll meet again in the morning for another exciting day of chair yoga.

CHAPTER TEN

THE YUMMY SIDE OF CHAIR YOGA

Mmm… can you smell it? The mouthwatering aroma of fresh fruit, the comforting warmth of a home-cooked meal, and the enticing sweetness of a piece of dark chocolate. Now, what if I told you that your next delicious meal could be the secret ingredient to enhancing your chair yoga practice? Yes, you heard it right. Your kitchen and your chair are about to become the best of buddies. So, grab a plate, pull up a chair, and let's discover the scrumptious world of chair yoga and nutrition!

Chair Yoga and Your Diet: A Match Made in Wellness Heaven

Balanced Meal Plans: Your Body's Fuel Gauge

Think of your body as a car. Your muscles are the engine, your breath is the accelerator, and your food is the fuel. Just like a car runs smoothly on the right kind of fuel, your body needs a balanced diet to function optimally.

A balanced meal plan should include a mix of macronutrients - carbohydrates for energy, proteins for muscle repair, and fats for brain health. A healthy balance of all of these macronutrients play a crucial part in the harmony of your health.

Here are a few tips to create a balanced meal plan:

- Fill half your plate with colorful fruits and vegetables. Let your plate look like a rainbow, each color providing a different set of nutrients.

- Choose lean proteins like chicken, fish, tofu, or beans. It's like selecting the building blocks for your muscles.

- Include whole grains like brown rice, quinoa, or whole wheat bread. They're your body's energy generators, providing slow-release carbohydrates to fuel your chair yoga practice.

- Don't forget healthy fats like avocados, nuts, seeds,

or olive oil. They're like the lubricant for your brain, keeping it sharp and focused.

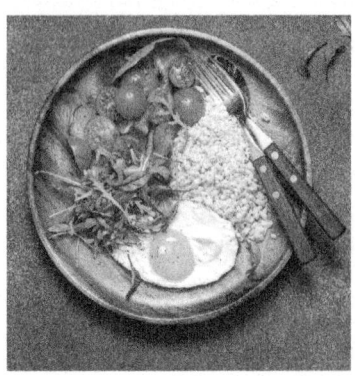

Hydration Importance: The River of Life

Now, let's talk about hydration, the river of life that keeps your body running smoothly. Imagine a garden without water. The plants would wither, the flowers would droop, and the soil would dry up. Similarly, without adequate hydration, your body can't function optimally.

Water plays a crucial role in digestion, nutrient absorption, temperature regulation, and even joint lubrication.

Here are a few tips to stay hydrated:

- Aim for at least 8 glasses of water a day. It's like setting a baseline, a starting point for your hydration goals.

- Drink a glass of water before and after your chair yoga practice. This preps your body for the session and replenishes it afterward.

- Keep a water bottle handy. When it is nearby, it's more accessible prompting you to take frequent sips throughout the day.

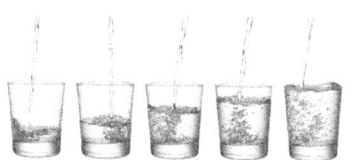

Snacking Right: The Art of Mindful Munching

Finally, let's talk about snacks, those delightful mini-meals we all love. Now, snacking can be a double-edged sword. On one side, it can provide you with a quick energy boost between meals. On the other, it can lead to overeating and weight gain.

The key lies in snacking right, choosing nutritious snacks that fuel your body without loading it with empty calories. It's like choosing the right accessories for your outfit, enhancing your look without going overboard.

Here are a few tips to snack right:

- Choose snacks rich in protein and fiber like yogurt, nuts, or fruits. They're like slow-burning candles, providing you with steady energy.

- Avoid sugary snacks that cause a quick spike and crash in your energy levels.

- Practice mindful eating, paying attention to your hunger and fullness cues. It's developing your unique conversation with your body, understanding its needs, and responding accordingly.

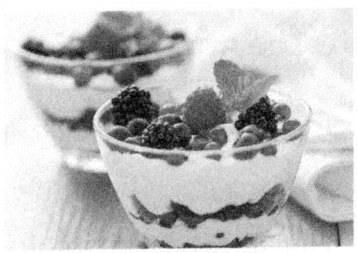

Now you have a guide to combining chair yoga with a balanced diet, adequate hydration, and mindful snacking. So, the next time you sit on your chair for a yoga session, remember that your kitchen can play a significant role in your fitness journey.

The Food-Yoga Connection: The Dynamic Duo

Foods for Flexibility: The Stretching Superstars

Did you know food and what you put on your plate can help you on your journey towards better flexibility?

Omega-3 fatty acids are your allies here. Present in fatty fish like salmon and mackerel, flaxseeds, walnuts, and chia seeds, these nutrients are like a magic potion for your joints, boosting their flexibility and reducing inflammation.

Next in line are foods rich in magnesium, nature's muscle relaxant. Spinach, almonds, black beans, and bananas are packed with this fantastic mineral. It's like having a personal masseuse for your muscles, gently kneading out the knots and tensions, helping you stretch a little further in each yoga pose.

Finally, don't forget to load up on water-rich fruits and vegetables like cucumbers, watermelon, oranges, and strawberries. Hydration plays a key role in maintaining the elasticity and flexibility of your muscles.

Energy-Boosting Foods: The Powerhouses of Pep

Imagine you are the owner of a high-performance car and you're ready to take this beauty for a ride down the freeway. Now, what kind of fuel would you fill your tank with? Sugary snacks and refined carbs are like low-grade fuel. They might give you a quick energy boost, but it's followed by a plunge that leaves you feeling sluggish and tired.

On the other hand, complex carbs found in whole grains, legumes, and starchy vegetables are your premium-grade fuel. They provide your body with a steady stream of energy, keeping you revved up through your chair yoga practice. Complex carbs are your reliable co-pilot, navigating you through the ebbs and flows of your energy levels.

Lean proteins like chicken, turkey, tofu, and Greek yogurt are also excellent energy boosters. Lean proteins are sturdy pillars holding up your structure and providing a solid foundation of energy that keeps you strong and steady.

Lastly, don't forget to sprinkle some seeds and nuts into your diet. Packed with healthy fats, they're like tiny batteries, storing energy for when you need it. Plus, they make a tasty topping for salads, yogurts, and even stir-fries!

Anti-Inflammatory Diet: The Pacifiers of Pain

Picture a calm, serene lake, its surface undisturbed by even a ripple. That's the state of peace and balance we want in our bodies, and an anti-inflammatory diet can help us get there.

Foods rich in antioxidants are your first line of defense. Berries, dark chocolate, artichokes, and even a glass of red wine (in moderation, of course!) are packed with these inflammation-fighting compounds.

Spices like turmeric and ginger not only add a zing to your dishes but also have potent anti-inflammatory properties. So spice is a protective shield in your meal, guarding your body against inflammation.

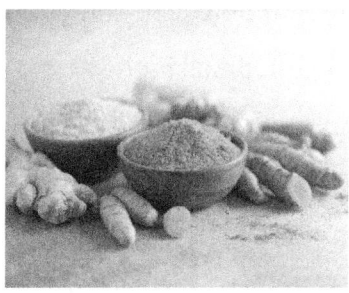

Fatty fish, walnuts, and flaxseeds are rich in Omega-3 fatty acids and are known for their anti-inflammatory effects.

The ideas shared are in no way exhaustive; however, they are a starting point. Let them be a guide to how the right foods can enhance your chair yoga practice, boost your flexibility, energize your body, and reduce inflammation. It's not just about the poses or the breathwork. It's about fueling your body with the right nutrients to support your chair yoga journey. So, the next time you step onto your chair for a yoga session, remember the role your kitchen plays in your fitness journey.

Your Plate, Your Yoga Mat: Savoring the Connection

Mindful Eating: Savoring Each Bite

Do you know that feeling of listening to your most loved song? It doesn't matter how many times you've heard it - every time you lose yourself in the moment. You're not just mindlessly humming along. You're savoring each note, each lyric, getting lost in the rhythm of the music. That's what mindful eating is all about - savoring each morsel, each flavor, immersing yourself in the experience of eating.

So, how do you eat mindfully? First off, ditch the distractions. Turn off the TV, put away your phone, and focus solely on your meal. Shine the spotlight of your attention on your food, letting it shine in all its glory.

Take the time to appreciate the look and smell of your food before you start eating. It's also taking a moment to be thankful.

Then, take small bites, chew slowly, and savor the flavor of each mouthful.

Pay attention to your taste buds and the sensations in your mouth.

Not only does mindful eating enhance your enjoyment of food, but it also helps you tune into your hunger and fullness cues, preventing overeating.

Food as Fuel: Powering Your Chair Yoga Practice

Now, let's shift gears and think of food as fuel for your chair yoga practice. Imagine your body now as that high-performance car. The food you eat is the premium fuel, propelling you towards your fitness goals.

Complex carbohydrates like whole grains, fruits, and vegetables provide you with sustained energy for your chair yoga sessions. It's like a long-lasting fuel that gives you energy to keep going.

Proteins from lean meats, dairy, and plant-based sources help repair and build muscles, supporting your strength and flexibility in chair yoga. Protein is the maintenance crew for your high-performance car, ensuring everything is in top shape for the journey.

Healthy fats from avocados, nuts, seeds, and oily fish provide essential fatty acids that support brain function, keeping you focused and alert during your practice. It's like the navigation system for your car, guiding you on your journey.

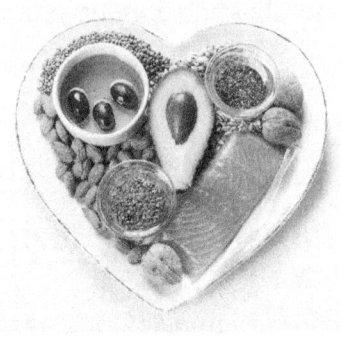

Nutrient Timing: The When of Eating

We've talked about the what and the how of eating. Now, let's address the when. Nutrient timing is all about coordinating your meals and snacks with your chair yoga practice to maximize energy and recovery.

Aim to have a balanced meal 2-3 hours before your chair yoga session. This gives your body enough time to digest the food and convert it into energy.

If you're practicing chair yoga first thing in the morning, a small snack 30 minutes before can give you a quick energy boost. Think of a banana, a piece of toast, or a yogurt.

After your chair yoga session, refuel your body with a mix of protein and carbohydrates to aid muscle recovery and replenish energy stores. It's like refueling your car after a road trip, preparing it for the next journey.

There you have it - a guide to mindful eating, viewing food as fuel, and the importance of nutrient timing with chair yoga. It's not just about what's on your plate or how you eat it; it's also about when you eat and how it aligns with your chair yoga practice. So, the next time you roll out your chair for a yoga session, remember that your diet plays a key role in your fitness journey. From your plate to your yoga mat, here's to a healthier, happier you!

Foods That Make Your Yoga Pose Better

Foods for Muscle Recovery: The Soothing Embrace

Have you ever felt that characteristic muscle soreness after a particularly engaging chair yoga session? That's your muscles telling you they've had a good workout and now need some tender loving care. And what better way to show them love than with the right foods?

Protein-rich foods are your muscles' best friends when it comes to recovery. When a bricklayer is building a brick wall, each brick lays the foundation for the next, creating a strong and sturdy structure. That's what proteins do for your muscles. They provide the building blocks, aiding in repair and growth after a workout. Foods like chicken, tofu, eggs, and Greek yogurt are all protein powerhouses.

Now, let's add some cherries to this nutritious mix. Cherries, especially tart ones, are known for their anti-inflammatory properties and can help reduce muscle soreness.

Pre-Yoga Foods: The Energy Sparklers

Now, let's talk about what to eat before your chair yoga practice. It's like fueling up your car before a road trip. You want to make sure you've got enough fuel to keep you going, but not too much that it weighs you down.

A light snack about an hour before your practice is a good idea. Bananas are a great choice. They're rich in fast-acting carbohydrates that provide quick energy and are also packed with potassium, which supports nerve and muscle function.

Another good option is a smoothie made with fruits and Greek yogurt. It's a tasty blend of carbs and proteins, providing sustained energy throughout your practice. It's like a melody of flavors, harmonizing to fuel your body.

Post-Yoga Foods: The Nourishing Hugs

Once you've completed your chair yoga practice, it's time to refuel your body. Here, you want a mix of proteins and carbohydrates. Proteins, as we saw earlier, help with muscle recovery. Carbohydrates, on the other hand, help replenish your energy stores. It's like giving your body a big, nourishing hug, thanking it for its hard work.

A post-workout meal could be something like a chicken wrap with lots of colorful veggies. It's a complete meal, providing protein from the chicken, carbs from the wrap, and a range of vitamins and minerals from the veggies.

Or, if you prefer something lighter, how about a bowl of oatmeal topped with nuts and berries? It's a comforting bowl of goodness, with carbs from the oats, protein from the nuts, and antioxidants from the berries.

The right foods can indeed make your chair yoga pose better, by fueling your body, aiding muscle recovery, and replenishing energy stores. Remember, your body is a temple, and food is the nourishment it needs to function optimally. Treat your body with love and respect, fuel it with nutritious food, and it will reward you with strength, flexibility, and wellness.

CHAPTER ELEVEN

BEGINNER'S AND SENIOR'S CHAIR YOGA

KEEPING THE FLAME ALIVE

The road to fitness is often peppered with ambitious goals, sweat-drenched workout clothes and, unfortunately, a pile of unused gym memberships. But what if we could swap this intimidating journey for a comfortable seat that leads us to wellness? With chair yoga, this dream becomes a reality. But how do we keep the excitement alive in this journey and make chair yoga a regular habit? That's exactly what we're about to explore, so let's get started!

How to Keep the Chair Yoga Fire Burning

Just like maintaining a campfire requires the regular addition of logs, maintaining the chair yoga fire in our lives requires consistent effort, realistic goals, and a hearty celebration of victories, small or large.

Setting Realistic Goals: The Roadmap to Success

When we talk about goals in chair yoga, it's not about touching your toes or perfecting a challenging pose. It's about setting achievable targets that make you feel good and motivate you to remain consistent.

Let's say you're a beginner who can practice chair yoga for 10 minutes without feeling tired. Instead of aiming to double this time in just a week, set a more realistic goal. Aim to add an extra 2-3 minutes to your practice each week. By setting manageable targets, you're more likely to stick to your practice and experience the many benefits of chair yoga.

Tracking Progress: The Joy of Growth

Seeing your progress is an instant morale booster and a great way to stay motivated. Remember, progress in chair yoga isn't just about losing weight or improving flexibility. It's also about feeling more energized, sleeping better, or even mastering a new pose.

Consider maintaining a chair yoga journal. After each session, jot down what poses you did, how long your practice was, and any changes you noticed in your energy levels or mood. Over time, flipping through this journal will give you a clear picture of your progress and inspire you to keep going.

Celebrating Small Wins: The Fuel of Motivation

In our journey of chair yoga, every small win counts. Maybe you held a pose for a few seconds longer, or perhaps you managed to practice chair yoga for five days in a row. These are all victories worth celebrating!

So how do we celebrate? It doesn't have to be a grand party. It could be treating yourself to a relaxing bath, spending an evening doing what you love, or simply acknowledging your achievement and giving yourself a pat on the back. When we celebrate our progress, we fuel our motivation to continue this journey.

Remember, the flame of chair yoga in our lives stays alive not by grand gestures, but by consistent effort, a positive mindset, and a whole lot of self-love. So, here's to setting realistic goals, tracking our progress, and celebrating every victory along the way! The chair awaits, and so does your journey towards wellness and joy.

Making Chair Yoga a Family Affair

Remember those chilly winter nights when the whole family would gather around the fireplace, sipping hot cocoa, sharing stories, and creating memories? Now, imagine adding a pinch of chair yoga to this cozy setting. Fun, isn't it? Here's how you can make chair yoga a cherished family affair.

Partner Poses: Double the Fun

It's time to ditch the solitary yoga sessions and invite a partner to join the fun. It could be your spouse, a sibling, or even a grandchild. The idea is to add some laughter, bonding, and a dash of friendly competition to your chair yoga routines.

Let's start with a simple pose: the Seated Twist. Sit back to back with your partner on your respective chairs. As you both inhale, sit up tall, lengthening your spine. On the exhale, twist towards your right, placing your right hand on the backrest of your chair and your left hand on your partner's knee. Your partner will do the same, and voila! You've nailed your first partner pose.

Next up is the Double Tree Pose. While seated, both of you lift your right knee and place your right foot on the inside of your left thigh. Now, reach out and hold each other's right hand, stretching your arms out to the side. It's like forming a small, charming forest right in your living room.

Fun Group Activities: The More, the Merrier

Why stop at partner poses? Let's extend the fun to the entire family. Get everyone together for an exciting session of chair yoga. You could even make it a part of your family gatherings or holiday traditions.

Begin with a simple group activity: the Seated Wave. Everyone sits in a circle on their chairs. The first person starts by raising their arms overhead, and then everyone else follows suit, one by one, creating a "wave" effect.

Another fun group activity is the Chair Yoga Train. Everyone forms a line, placing their hands on the shoulders of the person in front of them. The person at the front of the line leads the group through a series of chair yoga poses, with everyone following along.

Chair Yoga Games: Exercise in Disguise

If you've got kids or grandkids in the family, chair yoga games are a fantastic way to get them excited about exercise.

One simple game is Chair Yoga Simon Says. One person plays Simon and calls out different chair yoga poses. The rest of the group has to follow along, but only when the instruction starts with "Simon says".

Another fun game for the little ones is Chair Yoga Bingo. Create bingo cards with pictures of different chair yoga poses. Call out the poses one by one, and the players have to perform the pose and mark it on their cards. The first one to complete a row wins.

Chair yoga doesn't have to be a solo activity. By incorporating partner poses, group activities, and games, you can make it a fun-filled family affair. Not only will this spice up your routines, but it will also create a shared experience that brings everyone closer. So, pull up your chairs, gather your loved ones, and let the chair yoga fiesta begin!

When Life Gets in the Way of Chair Yoga

There's an old saying that "life is what happens when you're busy making other plans." It's true, life can sometimes throw a wrench in the best-laid plans, including our chair yoga routine. However, the beauty of chair yoga is its adaptability. It can slide into the busiest of schedules, like a bookmark tucked into a favorite novel, ready to be accessed anytime. So, let's explore how chair yoga can fit into your life, no matter how packed your schedule may be.

Quick Chair Yoga Routines: Fitness in a Flash

The clock ticks away, the to-do list grows, and before you know it, the day has sped past leaving no time for your chair yoga practice. Sounds familiar? When pressed for time, instead of skipping your practice altogether, why not opt for a quick chair yoga routine?

Here's a simple 5-minute routine that you can do anytime, anywhere:

- Start with a Seated Mountain Pose. Sit tall in your chair, feet flat on the ground, hands resting on your thighs. Take a few deep breaths, feeling your body grounding into the chair.

- Next, transition into a Seated Cat-Cow Stretch. Place

your hands on your knees. As you inhale, arch your back and lift your chest upwards. As you exhale, round your back and drop your chin towards your chest. Repeat this a few times, moving with your breath.

- Lastly, do a Seated Forward Bend. As you exhale, fold forward from your hips, letting your hands rest on your shins or the floor.

There you go! In just 5 minutes, you've stretched your spine, released tension from your body, and invigorated your senses.

Yoga During Commercial Breaks: Fitness Meets Entertainment

So you are vegging out and you're engrossed in your favorite TV show when suddenly, it cuts to a commercial break. Instead of reaching for your phone or fast-forwarding, why not use this break for a quick chair yoga session?

Start with a simple Seated Twist. As you inhale, lengthen your spine. As you exhale, twist your upper body to the right, placing your right hand on the backrest of your chair and your left hand on your right knee. Hold for a few breaths, then switch sides.

Next, try the Chair Eagle Pose. Extend your arms in front of you, cross your right arm over the left, bend your elbows and wrap your forearms around each other. Hold this pose till the commercial break ends, then unwind your arms and relax.

Voila! You've turned a commercial break into a mini yoga session. It's chair yoga meets entertainment!

Chair Yoga at Work: The Office Oasis

Imagine transforming your workspace into a mini yoga studio. Sounds intriguing, right? Chair yoga poses can easily be done at your desk, making them a perfect pick-me-up during a busy workday.

Start with the Chair Pigeon Pose. While seated, place your right ankle on your left knee, keeping your right knee relaxed. Hold this pose for a few breaths, feeling a gentle stretch in your right hip.

Next, try the Seated Crescent Moon Pose. Lift your arms overhead, interlace your fingers, and lean to your right, stretching your left side. Hold for a few breaths, then switch sides.

Lastly, close your eyes and take a few deep breaths, letting go of any stress or tension from your body. It's like a mini vacation, right at your desk.

So, there you have it. Whether you're pressed for time, engrossed in a TV show, or swamped with work, chair yoga can find its way into your schedule. It's flexible, adaptable, and always ready to fit into your day. Here's to chair yoga, your faithful companion in the bustling journey of life!

The Secret Sauce for Sticking to Chair Yoga

Consistency Over Intensity: The Tortoise's Tale

Remember the classic fable of the tortoise and the hare? The hare, fast and cocky, dashes off at top speed, while the tortoise, slow and steady, plods along at a consistent pace. And who wins the race? The tortoise, of course! This tale isn't just a bedtime story, it's a philosophy that applies beautifully to chair yoga.

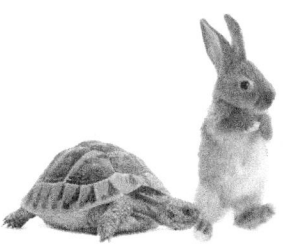

When it comes to chair yoga, it's not about how fast you can stretch or how many poses you can master in a week. It's about showing up on your chair, day after day, and being present in your practice. It's about the persistence of doing a little bit every day rather than pushing yourself too hard and burning out. It's the tortoise's secret to winning the race, and it could be yours too.

Variety in Routine: The Spice of Chair Yoga Life

Imagine eating the same meal day in and day out. No matter how delicious it is, you'd soon get bored, right? The same principle applies to chair yoga. Doing the same poses in the same order every day can turn your practice into a tedious chore rather than a joyful experience.

The beauty of chair yoga lies in its diversity. From the gentle Seated Forward Bend to the energizing Chair Sun

Salutation, there's a plethora of poses to choose from. You can experiment with different sequences, focus on different areas of your body, or even try new breathing techniques. You get to decide and have the freedom to pick and choose what you fancy. This variety keeps your practice fresh and exciting, enticing you to stick with it.

Enjoyment in Practice: The Chair Yoga Symphony

I'm a music lover and love the energy of being at a live concert. Do you know that feeling when the music resonates with your soul, the rhythm makes your body sway, and you lose yourself in the symphony. Now, imagine feeling the same way about chair yoga. Sounds wonderful, doesn't it?

Chair yoga isn't just a form of exercise, it's an experience. It's an opportunity to tune into your body, to explore its capabilities, and to appreciate its strength. When you start enjoying your chair yoga practice, it's no longer a task on your to-do list, it's a melody in the symphony of your day.

So, whether you're a beginner just testing the waters or a seasoned practitioner, remember the three vital ingredients to stick to chair yoga: consistency, variety, and enjoyment. It's not about pushing yourself to the limit, it's about weaving chair yoga seamlessly into the fabric of your life. It's about making chair yoga a part of your daily routine, just like brushing your teeth or having your morning coffee. And, most importantly, it's about enjoying the practice, about finding joy in every stretch, every breath, every moment on the chair.

As we continue our exploration of chair yoga, we'll delve into more poses, more techniques, and more fun ways to make this practice an integral part of your life. So, go ahead, pull up your chair, and let's keep this beautiful symphony playing. Your chair is waiting, and so is your journey to a healthier, happier you.

Chapter Twelve

Tales from the Chair

Real-life Victories with Chair Yoga

Have you ever found yourself amidst a crowd, all eyes on the stage, as one by one, people step up to the microphone and share their stories? Some stories inspire, some amuse, some tug at your heartstrings, but each one leaves an indelible imprint on you. That's what we're about to do in this chapter. We're going to pull up a chair, gather around, and share some remarkable stories of victories achieved through the magic of chair yoga. These are tales of transformation, tales of perseverance, tales of rediscovering oneself. So, grab a cup of tea, settle in, and let's delve into the heartwarming world of chair yoga testimonials.

Real-life Testimonials of Chair Yoga Victories

Weight Loss Triumphs: The Scale Doesn't Lie

Picture a lady in her late sixties, let's call her Mabel. Mabel had always struggled with her weight. The numbers on the scale seemed to only go one way - up. She had tried dieting, gym memberships, and even dance classes, but nothing seemed to stick. That's when she discovered Chair Yoga. At first, she was skeptical. Can sitting on a chair really help her lose weight? But she decided to give it a try.

Fast forward six months, Mabel had lost over 20 pounds! But it wasn't just about the numbers on the scale. She felt lighter, both physically and emotionally. She could move around more easily, do things she hadn't done in years. But the cherry on top? She had to go shopping for new clothes because her old ones were too big! Mabel's story is a testament to the potential of chair yoga as a tool for weight loss, gently guiding you toward your goal, one pose at a time.

Improved Mobility Stories: The Freedom to Move

Now, let's turn the spotlight to George. George is a lively gentleman in his early seventies with a passion for gardening. But arthritis in his knees had taken a toll on his mobility. He couldn't kneel to tend to his flowers, couldn't bend to pull out the weeds. He felt like a bird with clipped wings. Then, he was introduced to chair yoga.

Within a few weeks of regular practice, George noticed a significant improvement in his mobility. He could bend his knees without wincing in pain, and could reach for the low shelves without struggling. But the real victory came when he could finally kneel to plant a new rose bush in his garden. The joy on his face was priceless. Chair yoga had given him back his freedom to move, the freedom to enjoy his beloved garden.

Enhanced Energy Levels: The Power to Seize the Day

Finally, let's meet Laura. Laura is a vivacious lady in her late fifties who loves spending time with her grandkids. But she often found herself exhausted by midday, her energy levels dipping, making her miss out on the fun. That's when she decided to try chair yoga.

In just a few weeks, Laura noticed a significant boost in her energy levels. She no longer felt the need to take a nap after lunch. She could play with her grandkids all afternoon without feeling drained. Chair yoga had infused her with newfound energy, turning her days from weary to wonderful.

From Chair Potato to Chair Yogi: Swapping the Remote for Yoga Poses

Overcoming Sedentary Lifestyle: The Great Indoors to the Great Active

Picture a cozy armchair, a captivating television show, and a bowl of popcorn. Sounds like a perfect afternoon, doesn't it? Now, let's introduce Betty. Betty, a jovial lady in her early fifties, loved her afternoons just like this. Ah, the comfort of her favorite armchair and the charm of her beloved soap operas. But soon, Betty realized that her sedentary lifestyle was taking a toll on her health.

Betty heard about chair yoga from a friend. Dismissing her initial doubts, she decided to give it a shot. In her living room, right there in front of the television, Betty swapped her remote for yoga poses. She started practicing chair yoga during the commercial breaks, stretching a little, and flexing a little. Slowly but surely, she was chipping away at her sedentary lifestyle.

Increased Activity Levels: Chair Yoga or A Workout Disguised as Fun

Fast forward a few weeks, Betty was spending more time practicing chair yoga than watching television. She was moving more, sitting less. She found herself looking forward to the commercial breaks, eager to try a new pose or perfect an old one. Chair yoga had transformed her days from hours of inactivity to periods of light-hearted workouts.

But the best part? Betty was having fun. She was laughing as she fumbled through a pose, smiling as she stretched a bit further, and celebrating as she held a pose a second longer. Chair yoga had turned her activity levels up a notch, and she was enjoying every bit of it.

Enhanced Quality of Life: A New Chapter in the Book of Life

Six months down the line, Betty could see a remarkable change in her life. She was more active, more energetic, and most importantly, healthier. Her blood pressure levels had come down, her joint pain had reduced, and she was feeling more flexible and balanced.

But it wasn't just about the physical health benefits. Betty was happier. She had discovered a new hobby and was enjoying a sense of accomplishment from her progress.

Chair yoga had not only improved her fitness levels but also enhanced her overall quality of life.

And so, Betty went from being a chair potato to a chair yogi, thanks to the magic of chair yoga. She swapped the remote for yoga poses, the television show for a fitness routine, and the popcorn for a healthier lifestyle. And you know what? She wouldn't have it any other way.

So, what's your story going to be like? Are you ready to swap your chair potato lifestyle for a chair yoga routine? Remember, it's never too late to start, and every little step counts.

Your Success is Our Success

Reader's Feedback: The Echo of Progress

Imagine a quiet room suddenly filled with the resonating sound of applause, the bright echo of laughter, and the soft whisper of encouragement. That's what the feedback from my readers and clients feels like - a symphony of voices that adds color, texture, and depth to the chair yoga community.

I've received countless messages from readers and clients like you, sharing your experiences, your triumphs, and your challenges. Each feedback is a precious gem, shining with its own unique story.

Take, for instance, Martha, who shared how chair yoga has helped her manage her chronic back pain. Or Sam, who reported an improvement in his balance and flexibility after just a few weeks of practice. And let's not forget Lisa, who found the motivation to ditch her sedentary lifestyle and embrace a healthier, more active one, thanks to chair yoga.

Each feedback is a testament to the power of chair yoga, a confirmation that we're on the right path. But more importantly, each feedback inspires us all to strive harder, to make chair yoga more accessible, more enjoyable, and more beneficial for everyone.

Shared Victories: The Collective Triumph

Think of a team winning a championship. The players, the coach, the fans - everyone shares in the victory, celebrating the collective triumph. That's how it feels when I hear about your victories in chair yoga. Each victory, no matter how big or small, is a shared triumph, a cause for collective celebration.

Remember Jane, who finally managed to touch her toes after months of practice? Or Mark, who lost 10 pounds through chair yoga and a balanced diet? And how about Susan, who found relief from her arthritis pain thanks to regular chair yoga sessions?

Each victory fills me with joy and pride. So celebrate each victory, not just for the achievement itself, but for the effort, perseverance, and determination behind it.

The Magic of Perseverance in Chair Yoga

Overcoming Obstacles: The Hero's Path

You get to be the hero of an epic adventure. You're journeying through a mystical land, facing numerous challenges and obstacles on your path. Every hurdle and every setback is a test of your courage, your resilience, and your will to succeed. That's what your chair yoga adventure is like. Each difficulty you face, and each challenge you overcome, adds to your growth, your strength, and your determination.

Let's meet John. John is a cheerful gentleman in his late sixties with a love for painting. However, a recent shoulder injury had left him struggling with pain and limited mobility.

Picking up a paintbrush felt like a daunting task, let alone creating a masterpiece. But John refused to let his injury steal his joy of painting. He decided to give chair yoga a try.

In the beginning, it was hard. Every movement, every stretch felt like a mountain to climb. But John didn't give up. He listened to his body, modified the poses to suit his comfort, and took one day at a time. His shoulder protested, his muscles ached, but John persevered. He faced the obstacle head-on, determined to regain his mobility and get back to his beloved canvas.

Persistence Pays Off: The Power of Never Giving Up

Fast-forward a few months, John's persistence started paying off. His shoulder pain started subsiding, his mobility started improving, and he could hold a paintbrush without grimacing in pain. He was not just overcoming his obstacle, but transforming it into a stepping stone towards his goal.

John's tale is a testament to the power of persistence. He showed us that chair yoga is not a race, but a marathon. It's not about how quickly you reach your goal, but about never giving up, no matter how tough the journey gets. Every stretch, every breath, every moment on the chair is a step forward, a small victory to celebrate.

Long-Term Benefits: The Gift that Keeps on Giving

Today, John is back to his canvas, painting with the same passion and joy as before. But the benefits of chair yoga didn't stop at improving his shoulder mobility. Chair yoga gave him a new perspective on health and wellness.

He started sleeping better, his chronic back pain reduced, and he felt more energetic and happier. He discovered a sense of balance, both in his body and his mind. And the best part? He continues to practice chair yoga, reaping its benefits each day.

John's story shows us that the benefits of chair yoga are not just immediate, but long-lasting. The time and effort you invest in chair yoga today will reward you with health, happiness, and well-being for years to come.

So, next time you find yourself facing an obstacle in your chair yoga practice, remember this story. Remember that courage, determination, and perseverance is a choice. Remember that every challenge is an opportunity for growth, every setback a setup for a comeback. And remember, the magic of chair yoga lies not just in the poses, but in the perseverance, in the never-give-up attitude, in the will to keep going, no matter what. So, here's to you, the heroes of our chair yoga adventure, and here's to the magic of perseverance in chair yoga.

As the sun sets on our tales of triumph, we look forward to the dawn of a new day, filled with the promise of new stories, new victories, and new adventures in the wonderful world of chair yoga.

CHAPTER THIRTEEN

YOU'VE GOT QUESTIONS, WE'VE GOT ANSWERS

UNMASKING CHAIR YOGA

You know that feeling of curiosity, like an itch you just can't scratch? That nagging question in the back of your mind that you're just dying to know the answer to? That's how it often is with chair yoga for beginners and seniors. You're intrigued by the idea, but there's a whirlpool of questions swirling around in your head. Fear not, for we're about to dive in and fetch those answers for you. So, fasten your seatbelts as we take a joyride through the most frequently asked questions about chair yoga.

Your Burning Questions Answered

Ideal Duration for Chair Yoga: The Goldilocks Principle

When it comes to the ideal duration for a chair yoga session, the Goldilocks principle comes into play. It's about finding that "just right" length of time that is neither too short nor too long but is just right for your comfort and fitness level.

For beginners, a session of 15 to 20 minutes can be a good starting point. It's long enough to get a feel for the poses and reap some benefits, yet short enough to not feel overwhelming or exhausting. As you get more comfortable with the practice, you can gradually extend your sessions to 30 minutes or even up to an hour.

Remember, the key is consistency. It's better to practice for a shorter duration regularly than to have long sessions sporadically. It's like watering a plant - a little bit every day is better than flooding it once in a while.

Best Time for Practice: Dawn, Dusk, or Anytime in Between?

When should you practice chair yoga - as the rooster crows or when the stars twinkle? The beauty of chair yoga is that it can be practiced at any time of the day that suits you.

If you're an early bird, a morning session can be a great way to start your day, filling you up with energy and positivity. Picture yourself greeting the sunrise with a refreshing chair yoga sequence - sounds uplifting, doesn't it?

If you're a night owl, an evening session can be a fantastic way to wind down and prepare for a good night's sleep. Imagine trading your nightly news for a calming chair yoga routine - a peaceful end to the day, indeed!

The most important thing is to choose a time when you can be fully present, free from distractions, and able to focus on your practice. It's like setting a date with yourself, a special time dedicated to your well-being.

Dealing with Physical Limitations: The Art of Adaptation

One of the most common concerns about starting chair yoga is dealing with physical limitations. Whether it's a bad knee, a troublesome back, or a bout of arthritis, physical conditions can pose challenges. But here's where the magic of chair yoga shines - it's adaptable and inclusive.

The beauty of chair yoga lies in its flexibility (pun intended!). Each pose can be modified to suit your comfort and ability. Use props, change positions, or adjust the range of movement as needed. It's like tailoring a suit - you adjust the seams, tweak the fit, and make it work for you.

For instance, if a pose requires you to lift your arm overhead but you have a shoulder issue, you could lift your arm as high as is comfortable for you. The aim is not to mimic the pose perfectly but to find a version of the pose that benefits you without causing discomfort or pain.

Remember, chair yoga is not a competition. It's a personal journey towards wellness, and each body has its own unique path. So, embrace your body with all its quirks and celebrate what it can do, rather than focusing on what it can't. After all, it's your body, your rules, and chair yoga is here to support you every step of the way.

Chair Yoga: Myth vs Reality

Debunking Common Myths

In the vast ocean of fitness and wellness, chair yoga is like an island of tranquility and accessibility. However, as with any island, there are a few myths floating around it. Let's set sail and debunk some of these myths, bringing clarity to our chair yoga adventure.

Chair Yoga is Only for Seniors

This is a common misconception that needs to be set straight. While chair yoga is indeed a fantastic choice for seniors due to its low impact and adaptability, it is not restricted to them. Anyone, regardless of age, can benefit from chair yoga. Think of it as a universal remote, designed to work for everyone.

Chair Yoga Isn't a "Real" Workout

Often, people assume that because chair yoga is performed in a seated position, it might not provide as rigorous a workout as other forms of yoga. This is far from the truth. Chair yoga can be as gentle or as challenging as you want it to be. It's like a choose-your-own-adventure book, where you set the pace and intensity of your practice.

Chair Yoga Can't Help with Weight Loss

This myth is a bit like a stubborn stain that refuses to go away. The reality is, chair yoga can indeed support weight loss. While it may not burn calories as quickly as running a marathon, it provides a holistic approach to weight loss, improving flexibility, boosting metabolism, and promoting mindfulness. It's like a multi-faceted gem, offering a range of benefits that collectively lead to weight loss.

Facts about Chair Yoga

Now that we've debunked some myths, let's shine a light on some facts about chair yoga.

Chair Yoga is Accessible

One of the standout features of chair yoga is its accessibility. It's designed to be inclusive, making yoga accessible to those with mobility issues, chronic pain, or any other physical limitations.

Chair Yoga Improves Flexibility and Strength

Chair yoga is excellent for improving flexibility and building strength. The various poses target different muscle groups, stretching and strengthening them. It's like a tune-up for your body, keeping it running smoothly and efficiently.

Chair Yoga Enhances Mental Well-being

Chair yoga isn't just about physical fitness. It's also a powerful tool for enhancing mental well-being. The combination of gentle movements and mindful breathing helps reduce stress, improve focus, and promote a sense of peace and calm.

Misconceptions Cleared

Finally, let's clear up some misconceptions about chair yoga.

You Need a Special Chair for Chair Yoga

This is not true. You can practice chair yoga on any chair that is comfortable, stable, and allows your feet to touch the ground when seated. If the chair has armrests, that can be an added benefit for some stretches.

Chair Yoga is Time-Consuming

On the contrary, chair yoga can easily fit into your schedule. You can practice it during a work break, while watching TV, or even while waiting for your morning coffee to brew. It's like a pocket-sized book, ready to be enjoyed whenever you have a few spare minutes.

Chair Yoga Requires a Lot of Equipment

Contrary to this misconception, chair yoga doesn't require any special equipment or props. While certain poses may use props for support or comfort, most poses can be performed using just a chair.

So, there you have it. We've debunked the myths, highlighted the facts, and cleared the misconceptions about chair yoga. And, just like that, our chair yoga island is a little less mysterious and a lot more inviting. So, feel free to pull up a chair and set foot on this island of tranquility and wellness. The chair yoga adventure awaits!

Chair Yoga: The Rumor Mill

Addressing Controversies: The Whispers in the Wind

There are whispers in the wind, rumors that float around, casting shadows of doubt and confusion about chair yoga. One such rumor is that chair yoga is a watered-down version of "real" yoga, that it's not an authentic practice. This couldn't be further from the truth.

Chair yoga is as authentic and effective as any other style of yoga. It shares the same ancient roots and philosophy as every other yoga practice. It's akin to the many branches of a tree, each unique yet connected to the same trunk.

Another rumor that often makes the rounds is that chair yoga is only for those with injuries or physical limitations. It's seen as a 'Plan B' for those who can't do "real" yoga. Again, this is a misconception. Chair yoga is for everyone - young or old, fit or unfit, flexible or not.

Clearing Doubts: Shining the Light of Truth

Let's shine the light of truth and clear some doubts about chair yoga. A common doubt people have is about the safety of chair yoga. Is it safe to twist and turn in a chair? Won't I fall off?

Rest assured, chair yoga is designed with safety as a top priority. The poses are carefully crafted to be performed while seated or using the chair for support. Of course, it's always important to listen to your body and stay within your comfort zone.

Another doubt people often have is about the effectiveness of chair yoga. Can sitting and stretching really help me lose weight? The answer is a resounding yes! While chair yoga may not burn calories as quickly as, say, running or aerobics, it offers a holistic approach to weight loss. It promotes flexibility, builds strength, reduces stress, and encourages mindful eating. It's a multi-faceted and holistic practice that tackles weight loss from multiple angles.

Setting the Record Straight: Breaking Down the Walls of Misinformation

Finally, let's set the record straight and break down the walls of misinformation about chair yoga. There's a rumor that you need special clothes or equipment for chair yoga. The reality is, you don't need any fancy attire or props for chair yoga. All you need is a chair and comfortable clothes that allow you to move freely.

Another rumor that needs busting is that chair yoga takes a lot of time. In actuality, you can squeeze in a chair yoga session any time you have a few spare minutes. It can be a quick 10-minute routine in the morning, a few stretches during your lunch break, or a relaxing sequence before bed.

We've addressed the controversies, cleared the doubts, and set the record straight about chair yoga. It's time to bid farewell to the whispers in the wind, the shadows of doubt, and the walls of misinformation. With the light of truth guiding us, we can now fully embrace the wonderful practice of chair yoga. So, pull up a chair and let's embark on this exciting adventure together. After all, chair yoga is not just a practice, it's a way of life.

The Most Unusual Questions About Chair Yoga

Unexpected Queries: The Curious Cat Strikes Again

You know how a cat's curiosity often leads it to explore the most unusual corners? That's exactly what some of our chair yoga enthusiasts do. Their curiosity about this practice often leads to some truly unexpected questions.

One such query was from a gentleman named Fred, who asked, "Can I practice chair yoga on a rocking chair?" An interesting question, indeed. While a rocking chair might add an element of fun to your practice, it might not provide the stable support needed for chair yoga poses. So, unless you're an expert at balancing, it's safer to stick to a regular, non-rocking chair.

Surprising Facts: The Hidden Treasures of Chair Yoga

As we chart the waters of chair yoga, we often stumble upon surprising facts, like hidden treasures in an unexplored ocean. One such fact is the impact of chair yoga on mental health.

A curious yoga enthusiast, Helen, once asked, "Can chair yoga help improve my memory?" Surprisingly, the answer is yes. Chair yoga, much like other forms of yoga, combines physical poses with mindful breathing and meditation, all of which can help improve cognitive functions like memory and attention. So, while you're stretching and twisting on your chair, you're also giving your brain a healthy workout.

Interesting Discoveries: Striking Gold in the Chair Yoga Mine

The world of chair yoga is like a gold mine, full of interesting discoveries waiting to be unearthed. One such discovery is the versatility of chair yoga poses.

I once received a query from a lady named Alice, who asked, "Can I practice chair yoga poses on a plane?" An unusual question, but with an interesting answer. Chair yoga poses are designed to be performed while seated, which makes them perfect for situations where moving around is not an option - like on a plane. So, the next time you find yourself squished in a plane seat, why not try a gentle chair yoga stretch to ease that muscle tension?

As we continue to explore the fascinating world of chair yoga, I encourage you to let your curiosity guide you. Don't hesitate to ask questions, no matter how unusual or unexpected they might be. After all, the most interesting discoveries often come from the most unexpected questions.

Well, dear reader, we have reached the end of this chapter, but it's not the end of our journey. We've answered some burning questions, debunked myths, addressed controversies, and unearthed surprising facts and unusual queries. But remember, there's always more to learn, more to explore. So, as we turn the page to the next chapter, let's keep our minds open, our curiosity alive, and our enthusiasm for chair yoga burning bright.

CONCLUSION

Well, dear reader, we've reached the end of our chair yoga adventure together. Like a well-cooked meal, we've savored every morsel of this journey, chewed on every tidbit of information, and hopefully, digested a healthy dose of inspiration.

The Takeaway: Live Better with Chair Yoga

Chair yoga isn't just about striking a pose on a chair; it's about striking a balance in life. It's about turning your ordinary chair into a magic carpet that carries you on a journey towards better health, increased energy, and improved flexibility. And the best part? You don't need a fancy yoga mat, a pair of stretchy pants, or the flexibility of a rubber band. All you need is a chair, a sprinkle of determination, and a dash of humor.

Your Next Steps: Beyond Your Chair

So, where do you go from here? Is this the end of your chair yoga journey? Of course not! It's just the beginning. You've got your map (this book), your compass (your body), and your guide (yours truly, a nurse turned yoga instructor). The rest of the journey is up to you.

Start by incorporating chair yoga into your daily routine. Remember, it's not about how long you practice, but how consistent you are. Five minutes a day is better than an hour once a week.

Next, experiment with different poses. Don't limit yourself to the ones we've discussed in this book.

Finally, don't be shy about sharing your chair yoga adventures. Spread the word, recruit some buddies, and make chair yoga the talk of the town!

Keep Calm and Do Chair Yoga

Along the way, you might face some bumps. Maybe your cat decides to use your chair as a scratching post, or your grandkids claim it as their pirate ship. Maybe your body protests a certain pose, or your mind refuses to focus. When that happens, remember our mantra: Keep calm and do chair yoga. With each inhale, lift your spirits, and with each exhale, let go of the stress. Remember, every warrior pose you strike, every breath you take, you're getting stronger, healthier, and happier.

A Toast to Your Chair Yoga Journey

And now, as we close this chapter, let's raise a toast to your chair yoga journey. Here's to the chair that transformed from a piece of furniture into a fitness tool. Here's to the body that stretched, twisted, and embraced the joy of movement. Here's to the mind that learned to focus, relax, and find peace amidst chaos. And most importantly, here's to you, dear reader, for taking the first step towards a healthier, happier life.

So, go forth, unroll your chair, and let the chair yoga magic unfold. Remember, in the world of chair yoga, there are no limits, just poses to be explored. Keep calm, keep practicing, and keep laughing, because chair yoga is not just about living better, it's about living happier.

Until we meet again, keep bending, keep breathing, and keep being awesome!

About the Author

Heather was a nurse for 14 years and always had a passion for holistic health, bringing presence and the whole person into her nursing practice. Her passion in nursing truly was connecting to humans, hearing their stories, and offering healing and support.

Heather has been a yoga practitioner and instructor for even longer – 18 years. Her unique medical background blends beautifully with her yoga experience. Heather always had a soft spot for her geriatric clients from visiting them in the community to long-term care. She wanted to offer ways for people who were chairbound or people with mobility limitations to benefit from yoga. She is passionate about addressing the misconceptions about yoga and making it accessible for all ages, levels, and capabilities.

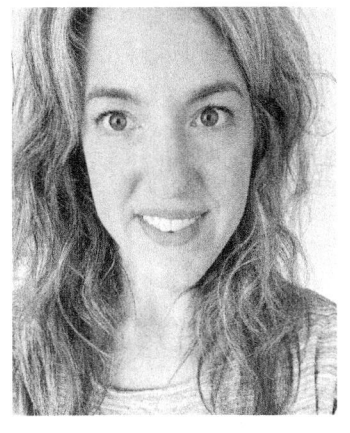

Underlying all of her work is her mission to live 'outside of the box', encourage daily movement as medicine, and raise awareness of the shame and taboos that exist in our society. She loves to dance and sing, spend time with her kids and pets, and explore her own healing with plant medicine. Heather is passionate about giving permission to men and women to release shame, bypass anxiety, be moved to make waves, come home to stillness, and BE RADIANT.

Heather loves to hear feedback from her readers.

Could you email her at info@heatheronhealth.com?

ALSO BY HEATHER DOLSON

BOOKS ON AMAZON AND AUDIOBOOKS ON AUDIBLE

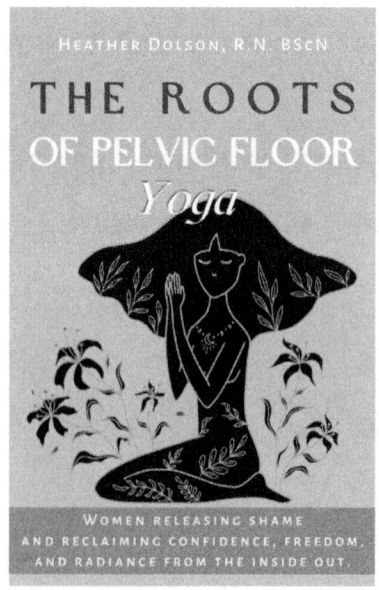

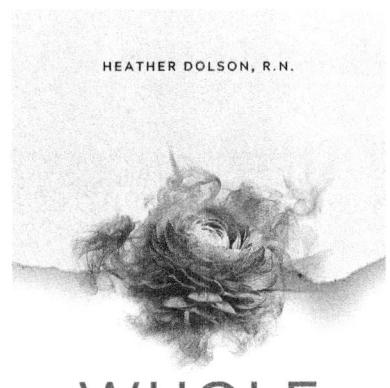

WHOLE

NAVIGATING THE TRAUMA
OF PREGNANCY LOSS

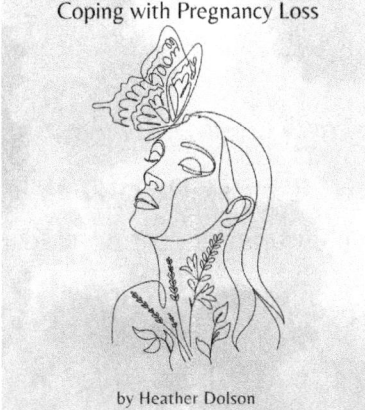

REFERENCES

Bonura, K. B., & Tenenbaum, G. (2014). Effects of yoga on psychological health in older adults. *Journal of Physical Activity and Health, 11*(7), 1334 -1341. https://doi.org/10.1123/jpah.2012-0365

Cho, S. T., & Kim, K. H. (2021). Pelvic floor muscle exercise and training for coping with urinary incontinence. *Journal of Exercise Rehabilitation, 17*(6), 379 – 387. https://doi.org/10.12965/jer.2142666.333

Food Surveys Research Group: USDA ARS. (n.d.). https://www.ars.usda.gov/northeast-area/beltsville-md-bhnrc/beltsville-human-nutrition-research-center/food-surveys-research-group/

Godman, H. (2023, June 1). *Harvard-led study: Yoga fights frailty.* Harvard

Health. https://www.health.harvard.edu/staying-healthy/harvard-led-study-yoga-fights-frailty

Grabara, M., & Szopa, J. (2015). Effects of hatha yoga exercises on spine flexibility in women over 50 years old. *Journal of Physical Therapy Science, 27*(2), 361–365. https://doi.org/10.1589/jpts.27.361

Kang, K. (2015). Effects of core muscle stability training on the weight distribution and stability of the elderly. *Journal of Physical Therapy Science, 27*(10), 3163–3165. https://doi.org/10.1589/jpts.27.3163

Leite, T. B. (2017). *Effects of different number of sets of resistance training on flexibility.* PubMed Central (PMC). https://www.ncbi.nlm.nih.gov/pmc/articles/PMC5609666/

López-Pérez, M. P., Afanador-Restrepo, D. F., Rivas-Campo, Y., Hita-Contreras, F., Del Carmen Carcelén-Fraile, M., Castellote-Caballero, Y., Rodríguez-López, C., & Aibar-Almazán, A. (2023). Pelvic floor muscle exercises as a treatment for urinary incontinence in postmenopausal women: A Systematic review of randomized controlled trials. *Healthcare, 11*(2), 216. https://doi.org/10.3390/healthcare11020216

Nazarpour, S., Simbar, M., Majd, H. A., & Tehrani, F. R. (2018). Beneficial effects of pelvic floor muscle exercises on sexual function among postmenopausal women: a randomized clinical trial. *Sexual Health*, *15*(5), 396. https://doi.org/10.1071/sh17203

Park, J., & McCaffrey, R. (2012). Chair Yoga: Benefits for Community-Dwelling Older Adults with Osteoarthritis. *Journal of Gerontological Nursing*, *38*(5), 12–22. https://pubmed.ncbi.nlm.nih.gov/22533347/

Physical activity for healthy aging. (2023, July 6). Centers for Disease Control and Prevention. https://www.cdc.gov/physicalactivity/basics/older_adults/index.htm

Saus-Ortega, C., Sierra-García, E., Martínez-Sabater, A., Chover-Sierra, E., & Ballestar-Tarín, M. L. (2023). Effect of pelvic floor muscle training on female sexual function: A systematic review protocol and meta-analysis. *Nursing Open*, *10*(9), 5790–5796. https://doi.org/ 10.1002/nop2.1826

Sharma, M., & Haider, T. (2012). Yoga as an alternative and complementary therapy for patients suffering from anxiety. *Journal of Evidence-Based*

Complementary & Alternative Medicine, 18(1), 15–22. https://doi.org/10.11772156587212460046

The effect of a yoga intervention on physical and psychological outcomes in patients on chronic hemodialysis. (2022, August 1). PubMed. https://pubmed.ncbi.nlm.nih.gov/36054806/

Weiss, C. (2021, January 4). *Mayo Clinic Q and A: Hot yoga for weight loss and overall health*. Mayo Clinic News Network. https://newsnetwork.mayoclinic.org/discussion/mayo-clinic-q-and-a-hot-yoga-for-weight-loss-and-overall-health/

Wersebe, H., Lieb, R., Meyer, A., Hofer, P. D., & Gloster, A. T. (2018). The link between stress, well-being, and psychological flexibility during an Acceptance and Commitment Therapy self-help intervention. *International Journal of Clinical and Health Psychology, 18*(1), 60–68. https://doi.org/10.1016/j.ijchp.2017.09.002

Woodyard, C. (2011). Exploring the therapeutic effects of yoga and its ability to increase quality of life. *International Journal of Yoga, 4*(2), 49. https://doi.org/10.4103/0973-6131.85485

Yao, C., Lee, B., Hong, H., & Su, Y. (2023). Effect of Chair Yoga Therapy on Functional Fitness and Daily Life Activities among Older Female Adults with Knee Osteoarthritis in Taiwan: A Quasi-Experimental Study. *Healthcare, 11*(7), 1024. https://www.ncbi.nlm.nih.gov/pmc/articles/PMC10094373/#:~:text=Findings%20from%20two%20intervention%20studies,osteoarthritis%20%5B11%2C25%5D.

Yoga for Pain: What the Science says. (n.d.). NCCIH. https://www.nccih.nih.gov/health/providers/digest/yoga-for-pain-science

BONUS RESOURCES

I have included two QR codes that you can scan with your phone.

You will be directed to 15-minute YouTube videos that can support you with your chair yoga practice. These are private videos I have made for my clients. Enjoy!